A Psychiatrist's English Training Manual

大慌て！精神科医ひろこ先生の
英語で診療・練習帳

ひまわりメンタルクリニック院長

小林博子 著

HIROKO KOBAYASHI , M.D.

JN064495

目次　CONTENTS

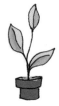

第三章 ちょっといい話 HANDY HINTS　*79*

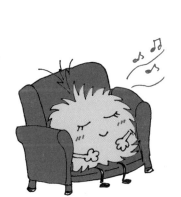

英語監修

Bret Prescott Fisk（ブレット　プレスコット　フィスク）

小説家、翻訳家。1972 年アメリカ合衆国生まれ。ユタ州とカリフォルニア州で育ち、1991 年に初来日。倫理学や日米関係史に興味をもち、様々な歴史問題に取り組んでいる。第二次世界大戦の歴史資料を二か国語で提供するウエブサイト『日本空襲デジタルアーカイブ』（http://www.japanairraids.org）を設立し運営。著書に『潮汐の間』・『紅蓮の街』（現代思想新社）、翻訳本に『 The Kazakh Khanates between the Russian and Qing Empires』（Brill社）などがある。英会話教室『Fisk English School 』（www.fiskenglishschool.com）経営。

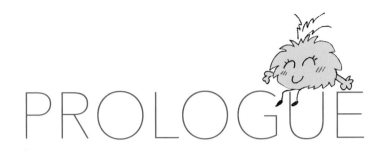

PROLOGUE

はじめに

この本は、
毎日英語で診察している方へというよりも、
時々英語で診察するような
機会があるかもしれないし、
日本語だったら、
もちろん口八丁手八丁、
いろいろ工夫して説明できるのに、
「はて？ 英語で
（日本語を母国語としない方へ）
どううまく伝えたらいいんだろう？」
と思う私のような方が
こっそり参考にできるものがあるといいな、
という趣旨で書かれたものです。
ですので、
自分が英語で診察している場面を想像して、
楽しんで読んでくだされば
幸いです。

Why have I written this book?

Why have I pushed myself to finish writing it?

Why is a psychiatrist who has never lived in an English-speaking country eager to engage in face-to-face English communication with non-Japanese patients?

Why don't I just use the type of portable translating machines that have already been adopted by many hospitals in Japan?

I can give you four reasons.

First, many people in the world speak English, making it a convenient means of communication even when it is spoken as a second language. Of course, Spanish and Chinese are also spoken by many people. At present, however, English is still the best choice for international communication.

Second, speaking English shows consideration for the feelings of those who have come to Japan but can't speak Japanese well yet. It is quite easy to imagine how helpless they must feel when they become sick in a foreign country. Some might say, "Do as the Romans do. If they come to Japan, they should learn to speak Japanese." That might be true. However, we must step forward and engage with them ourselves if they don't speak Japanese yet.

Here I would like to share a personal anecdote. Many years ago, I went to Germany as a graduate student. Just after arriving, I needed to have a medical checkup in order to receive a German grant I had applied for. For this reason, I visited a local physician even though I could hardly speak German. She gazed into my eyes gently and asked me several questions in English. I was very relieved and grateful for her kindness. At that moment I felt glad that I had come there. This personal experience is one of my main motivations for writing this book.

Third, please imagine the following situation. If I used a portable translating machine, I would have no choice but to sit and wait awkwardly while it spoke beside me. How should I spend those few moments? All I could do is make a troubled facial expression or smile unnaturally. How stupid I must look! Much better to communicate in English by myself, even if my English isn't perfect.

Fourth and last, writing this book will help me see patients in English. This book will serve as my own English training manual above all, but I hope others will also find it useful in their own daily practice.

Instead of dreading English study, I hope we can actually enjoy learning to communicate well with our patients and that this will lead to better diagnoses!

Within psychiatric treatment, it is very important to observe the patient's attitude and manner of answering questions. One must not only focus on speaking in English, but must analyze the patient carefully. English ability allows the doctor to relax and focus on what is important. Preparation is key! "Hope for the best, prepare for the worst!"

そうなのです。

「備えあれば憂いなし」です。

精神科では

「答えている患者さんの観察」も

大変重要ですから、

英語での質問に気を取られてばかりでは

いけないのだと思います。

なるべく心に余裕をもって

情報収集したいものですね。

私も大慌てで勉強し、

診療の準備をしているところですが、

取るものもとりあえず、

やってみましょう。

ここに記載されている英語は

アメリカご出身の日本語も堪能で

翻訳も手掛けている

Bret 先生監修ですので、

安心してお読みください。

●

ひまわりメンタルクリニック院長

小林博子

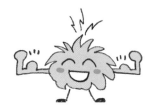

CHAPTER

第一章

総論

GENERAL REMARKS

初診予約から診察まで

最初の出会いは初診予約の電話から

　精神科診療を受けたいと思ったとき、患者さんまたはご家族は、いろいろなことを乗り越えて、すごく勇気をふり絞って、まず医療機関に電話をします。その時に、感じよく、丁寧な応対をされたら、患者さんはとても安心感をもてると思うのです。「そんなあなたを大切にします」という気持ちを込めて取り組んでいきましょう。

　One should never forget the importance of the initial contact with the patient. Psychiatric treatment begins from the first appointment call. It is often very hard for patients and their families to decide to see a psychiatrist, so, out of respect for their bravery, all clinic staff members should welcome them whole-heartedly and maintain a nice tone of voice, a positive attitude and emotional control.

　All visits to my clinic are made by appointment, so the first contact is always made by the receptionists answering the phone.

　私のクリニックは、英語対応医療機関ということになっていますが、小さな町の診療所です。受付事務の方にあまりストレスをかけるわけにもいかず、すべての事務の方が英語対応できるという現状でもなく、今のところは基本フレーズを提示し、それに従って電話を院長である私に回してもらう体制で行っています。

初診予約電話での会話

Patient : Hello.

Receptionist : This is Himawari Mental Clinic. Would you like to make an appointment for the first time? I'm sorry that we have no time available today. Advance reservations are needed. Another staff member will call you back later, so can I have your name and your phone number, please?

Patient : Oh, I see. My name is Tom Vector. My phone number is 090-XXXX-XXXX.

Receptionist : How do you spell your last name?

Patient : It's V as in victory, and e-c-t-o-r.

Receptionist : All right. Let me repeat that. 090-XXXX-XXXX. Is that OK?

➡ こんなことも聞かれるかもしれません。

Patient : What are your office hours? ── 診療時間はいつですか。

Receptionist : Our clinic hours are 9am to 3pm on Tuesday and Thursday. We are open 9am to noon on Wednesday and Friday. ── 火曜と木曜は午前9時から午後3時、水曜と金曜は午前9時から12時です。

Patient : Where exactly is the clinic? ── 場所はどこですか。

Receptionist :The closest train station is Kamonomiya. Kamonomiya is on the Tokaido line next to Odawara station. Only local trains stop there. Take the north exit, and it's a ten-minute walk from the station. If you don't want to walk, you can take a taxi. ── 東海道線の鴨宮駅が最寄り駅です。北口から歩いて10分です。タクシーもあります。

予約を確定するのに、再びこちらから電話連絡をします

Doctor : Hello. This is Dr. Hiroko Kobayashi. May I speak with Mr. Vector, please? Is this a convenient time to talk? The earliest available appointment for your first visit is Thursday June 5th at 12 o'clock. Is that OK for you?
—— 医師の小林です。ベクターさんですか。今お電話よろしいですか。予約は一番早くて6月5日12時からとなりますが、ご都合いかがでしょうか。

Doctor : The examination will take about one hour. You might have to wait a bit, if we are crowded that day.
—— 診察は1時間くらいです。混んでいるときはお待たせすることがあるかもしれません。

Doctor : Do you have a health insurance card? If not, you will have to pay the full fee in cash.
—— 保険証はお持ちでしょうか。そうでないと現金で10割負担となります。
We will be waiting for you at 12 o'clock on June 5th, Mr. Vector.
—— それでは6月5日12時にお待ちしています、ベクターさん。

> We look forward to seeing you at … でもいいかも、とBret 先生に言われました。私は「病気かもしれないと思ってクリニックを訪れる人に楽しみにしているようなこと言っておかしくない?」と確認したら、丁寧に話すなら問題ないと言われました。心情的に私には難しいと感じました。

➡ もしご家族からの電話だった場合
Staff : Could you tell me the patient's name and age, please?
—— 患者さんのお名前と年齢を教えていただけますか。

➡️ こんな時どうしよう？

当院はクレジットカードや小切手、トラベラーズチェックの対応をしていないので……

Patient : Do you accept credit cards? —— クレジットカードは使えますか。
Do you accept personal checks?

Staff : I'm sorry. We only accept cash, not credit cards or travelers' checks. —— 申し訳ありませんが、現金対応となっています。

Patient : May I pay in dollars/ euros/ pesos/ etc.?

Staff : I'm afraid you have to pay in Japanese yen. We can't accept dollars. —— 申し訳ありませんが、日本円だけでドルは使えません。

➡️ または…こんな時どうする？

お支払いの場所で、お金とか保険証を今日忘れたのですが……と言われても、きちんと伝えるべきところは伝えなければなりませんね。

Problem #1

Patient : I don't have any money with me now, but I can go home and get it. —— 今はお金の持ち合わせがないのですが、家にあるので取ってきます。

Problem #2

Patient : I'll be sure to bring my insurance card next time. So please let me pay the discounted rate from today. —— 次回必ず保険証を持ってきますので、今日も負担分を差し引いてもらえますか。

Staff : I'm sorry, but we can't do that. Please understand that we must follow regulations. However, you can get refund from your insurance later. —— 申し訳ありません。規則なものですから。でも保険会社から返金されると思います。

いかがでしょうか？

Staff : Hello, Mr. Vector. Here is a registration form for you to fill out. Please write your full name here. Bellow that, please write your home address and telephone number. Please give us your birthday, too. Write the year first, then the month and the day here.

Staff : Could you show me your health insurance card?
—— 保険証を見せていただけますか。

Staff : Also please fill out this questionnaire as much as you can.
—— この質問用紙にご記入ください。

Staff : Please take a seat in the waiting room.
—— どうぞおかけになってお待ちください。

待合室には静かなクラシック音楽が流れています。

呼ばれるまでのわずかな時間でも

ゆっくり過ごしてもらいたいものです。

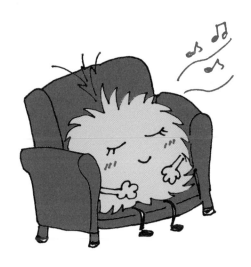

診察室にて〜
出会いは安心感から

「いろいろと立ち入ったことをお聞きしないとならなくて、ごめんなさいね。でもここでお話したことはどこにも漏れたりしませんから、安心していてくださいね」というようなことを言ってさしあげたいと思います。

Doctor : Please come in, Mr. Vector. I'm Dr. Kobayashi. I'm afraid that I have to start by asking you many personal questions. If you feel uncomfortable about anything or don't want to answer, please let me know. Rest assured that anything you tell me in our discussions will be kept confidential. So, how can I help you?

── ベクターさん、お入りください。小林といいます。個人的な質問もいたしますが、もし嫌だったら、おっしゃってくださいね。ここでお話しされたことはどこにも出ませんから（守秘義務）ね。さて、どうされましたか。

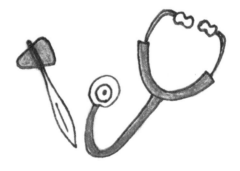

精神的症状の所見として

（根ほり葉ほりお聞きします）

❶ 睡眠について

● Can you sleep well?

　── 熟眠感はありますか？

● Can you fall asleep quickly?

　── 入眠障害は？

● If you wake up in the night, can you fall asleep again without trouble?

　── 中途覚醒からの入眠は？

● Do you wake up at the same time every morning?

　── 生活リズムは？

● Have you been waking up earlier or later than usual recently?

　── 早朝覚醒や過眠は？

❷ 食欲について

● Do you feel nauseous today?

　── 今日は吐き気とかしませんか？

● Do you sometimes feel like vomiting?

　── 吐きそうな感じはありますか？

● At these times do you actually vomit?

　── 本当に中身が出ることはありませんか？

● Can you keep your food down after eating?

　── 吐くことなく食べられていますか？

● Do you have an appetite?

　── 食欲は？

● Do you enjoy eating?

　── お食事、楽しめていますか？

● Do you look forward to eating？
　── あ〜♡お腹すいた!!と思いますか？
● Do you think of eating as a chore＊？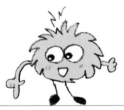
　── なんだか義務として食べていませんか？

> ＊choreという単語は辞書で引くと「家事・雑用」と出てきますが、単語のもつニュアンスとしてはネガティブな感じにやらなくてはならないことだそうで、ここでは「義務的に」というのにはこの単語がぴったりだそうです。

❸ 好きなことについて？

● What are your favorite things to do？
　── 何かお好きなこと、ありますか？
● For example, what are your hobbies？
　── 例えばご趣味とか？

質問用紙を見て……あなたの楽しみは○○と書いてありますが、

● Can you still enjoy them as much as you used to？
　── 以前のように楽しめていますか？

　これらはやはり、患者さんの答えるしぐさや雰囲気、視線の動きなど診断の参考になりますので、患者さんのご負担にならない範囲でさらりと聞けるといいですね。質問をする私のほうが緊張しないことが大切かもしれませんけど。

> 患者さんへの相づちの打ち方として、「わかりました」というのは、
> I understand.
> と現在形で答えるのがいいそうです。日本語に引きずられて過去形にしないよう注意が必要です。

身体所見と神経学的所見

初診時では、身体所見と神経学的所見をきちんと取らなくてはなりません。医学生のころ、「精神科を希望している学生は身体所見を、身体科に行きたい学生は精神学的所見をおろそかにしてはいけません」と言われたことが、今、身に染みて感じます。本当にそうなのですよね。

A physical examination can be an important component when assessing the condition of a patient presumed to have a psychiatric illness. Knowledge of the basics of neurologic examination, especially those components that are effective in screening for neurologic dysfunction, is essential for all clinicians, including, of course, psychiatrists.

それでは、いつも初診時に行っている身体所見・神経学的所見を英語でスムーズに取ってみましょう。

◎ 嗅神経について

● I'm going to put something fragrant in front of your nose.
Please close your eyes and sniff it, then tell me what it is.

In my clinic, I use mild smells, such as toothpaste, coffee or curry.
ちなみに私のクリニックでは、ペパーミント歯磨き粉とインスタントコーヒーそしてカレー粉を使用しています。皆さんのところはいかがされてますか？

◎ 眼について
（対光反射）

● I'm going to use my pen light to examine your pupils. I know it is hard but please try to keep your eyes open until I'm finished. It will only take a few seconds.

結構まぶしいけど、ごめんなさいね、頑張って！ という気持ちで。

（目の動きをみる）

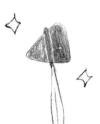

● Can you see the head of this hammer?

当院ではハンマーを目で追ってもらっています

● Does it look normal or do you have double vision?

（I mean "can you see it as a single object?"）

Now I will move this hammer slowly in front of your face.

Please follow it with your eyes only. Don't move your head.

または Please keep your head as still as you can and follow this hammer

with your eyes.

ここで、目の動きばかりでなく、言葉への理解力も知れるところなので、落ち着いてきちんと指示できることが大事だと思います。

◎ 舌について

● Open your mouth and say, "Ah."（舌の奥の咽頭をみる）

● Open your mouth and show me your tongue.（舌の動きを確認する）

Stick out your tongue as far as possible.

── できるだけ舌を出してみてください。

Please move your tongue from side to side.

── 左右に舌を動かしてみてください。

◎ 味覚について

● Do you have any difficulty in tasting your food?

── 味はわかりますか？

● Does it taste bitter when you eat something sweet?.

── 甘いものが苦く感じることはありませんか？

● Have you ever felt like you were biting sand or cardboard when you

were eating something?
—— 砂や段ボールを噛むように感じたことはありますか？

◎ 体温・血圧測定

● I'd like to check your lungs and heart now.（聴診のとき）
● I'm going to take your temperature.（体温測定のとき）
  Keep this thermometer under your arm.
● Let me measure your blood pressure and pulse.（血圧測定のとき）
  Please don't talk while I measure it.
  Can you roll your sleeves up to here?
  （上腕くらいの「ここら辺」までまくってください、と指示を出す）
  I'm going to wrap this cuff (Manchette) around your arm.
  It will get a little tight, but please don't be afraid.
  If you feel any pain, please tell me.
これは特に認知症の方など〜血圧測定の理解が困難な方〜に話をする感じ
を想定しています。

◎ 手の観察

● Spread your fingers open as wide as possible.
  —— 手をできるだけピーンと広げてください。

During this examination, we should observe the patient's fingernail
condition and palm color, and as well as check for any sweating.
手を広げている間に爪の状態、手掌の変化・発汗など診られますので注意
して観察しましょう。
● Do your hands shake?
  —— 震えませんか？

● Have you ever noticed your hand trembling while eating or handling small objects?
　―― 食事や細かい作業で震えを感じたこと、ありますか？

正確な指示ができてこそ正確な所見が取れるのだと思います。身振り手振りも有効に使いながら、頑張っていきましょう。

● Please do this!　（こんなふうにお願いします）
● Please copy what I'm doing with my hand!
● my hand / my arm / my leg などなど
と、私がやって見せて、こんな感じで！ というのもありだと思います。

◎ Rapid Alternative Movement では手首の回内、回外を急速に繰り返す
（反復拮抗運動試験）

● Move your hands on your knees as fast as you can like this.
とやって見せる。
● "That's perfect! Can you go faster?"（と応援しましょう）
そして "Thank you. Great job!"（ありがとうございます。お疲れさまでした）

◎ Finger-Nose-Finger Exam. の時は（指鼻試験）

● Using your index finger, touch your nose and then touch my index finger, and then touch your nose again like this.

◎ Walking Exam. 歩行を調べる時も（tangem gait・つぎ足歩行）
● Can you see the straight line on the floor?
● Please walk on the straight line heel-to-toe like this.
　（自分で手本を見せる）

● I'll be here to help you if you lose your balance.

倒れそうになったら、私が支えますから、と安心感を与えてから行いましょう。

◎ 深部腱反射　**Deep Tendon Reflexes**

● I'm going to examine your tendon reflexes with this hammer.

　または

　I'm going to tap your knee with this hammer to check your reflexes.

　Do you have any knee pain today?

高齢女性には膝痛のある方が多いので、注意・確認しましょう。

● If not, we'll start the exam now. Please stay relaxed.

　Please try to relax and let your arms rest on your lap.

Actually, it is very difficult to voluntarily relax for people who feel nervous, so please start by flexing then relaxing your arm.

緊張の強い患者さんでは力を抜けと言われても、難しいことが多いので、一回ギューッと力を入れてもらってからバーンと抜く方がうまく検査できることが多いですね。

◎ 血液検査

● Have you ever had negative results on a blood test related to anemia, liver dysfunction, hyperlipidemia, etc?

　── 今まで、貧血・肝機能・脂質異常症など異常を指摘されたことはありますか？

● How long ago did you take that exam?

　── それは何年前ですか？

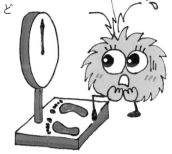

認知機能検査

　私はこの検査が大好きです。検査をしているときのしぐさや態度を見させてもらうのがとても大切なことなので認知機能検査は焦ることなく行いましょう。また、時事ネタとか最近のニュースなどをさりげなく聞けるとなおいいですね。

　「物忘れとか気になることはありますか？」とお聞きして、もし少しでもあると答えれば「それではいい機会ですから、一度どのくらい物忘れしているのか、調べさせていただけませんか？」と言い、反対に、ないとおっしゃれば「65歳以上の方には、皆さんにやっている試験ですので、ご協力お願いします。簡単なこともお聞きするかもしれませんが、お許しくださいね」と導入しています。

　そして、患者さんを励ます言葉を使いたいです。言葉はある意味パワーをもっていますから。医療者の心無い一言で傷つけないようにしたいものです。

　それでは、いつも初診時に行っている身体所見・神経学的所見を英語でスムーズに取ってみましょう。

　I really like the HDS-R cognitive examination and I find it very useful. Because it is so important to carefully observe the patients' gestures and attitude during the examination, I always try to conduct them in detail but without being nervous. In addition, it seems much helpful to mix up the examination questions with current topics and news.

　Before starting the exam, I always ask my patients this question. "Do you ever feel forgetful?"

　If they answer "yes", I say something like "Oh, great. This will be a good opportunity to talk about anything worrying you in your daily life."

If they answer "no", I reply "I see. That's good! On the first visit I always have to ask these questions. I'm afraid it might be too easy for you, but let me begin now. Are you ready?" Especially when working with elderly people who are often anxious about their memory, I want to encourage them and give them hope by using positive words. Doctors should always remember the power their words have to either encourage or injure the hearts of their patients.

Let's begin.（さあ、始めましょう）

---

1. 今日は何年何月何日ですか?

● What's the date today?
● Do you know the year? What month is it?
You can look at this calendar, if you like.
と助け船を出してもいいですね。

---

2. 今日は何曜日ですか?

● What day is it today?
● What day of the week is it?

---

3. おいくつですか?

● Could you tell me how old you are?
　How old are you, Ms. Garden?
確かに長い文の方が丁寧ですが、疑問文は話すイントネーションにより印象がかなり違うので、下の文でもゆっくりきちんと言えば、ポジティブな意味でどちらでもいいようです。

4. 私が言う言葉を繰り返してください（3 つの言葉）

● Please repeat each word after me.

Tulip ⇒ Dog ⇒ Car

Please remember these three words. I'll ask you to tell them to me again in a few minutes.

「私のあとについて繰り返してください。あとで聞きますから覚えておいてください」。日本語では皆さんもよくご存じのように桜 ⇒ 猫 ⇒ 電車ですが、チューリップを入れてみました。これは皆さんの創意工夫で！ お願いします。

★ 次の **test** に移るとき：Are you ready for the next thing?

5. 100 から 7 を順番に引き算してみてください

● I want you now to count backward by 7's from 100.

Let's subtract in a series of seven starting from 100.

Please calculate like this.

100 − 7 = ?　What is 100 minus 7?

100 minus 7 is?

途中でつっかかっても keep going！と応援しましょう。

6. 数字を逆に言ってください（数字の逆唱）

「これから言う数字を逆に言ってください。例えば、1 ⇒ 2 ⇒ 3 と私が言ったら、逆から 3 ⇒ 2 ⇒ 1 というように答えてください。それでは、6 ⇒ 8 ⇒ 2 は？」

● Let's go to the next question.

Please reverse the order of the following numbers. For example, 1-2-3 becomes 3-2-1. OK? So, how about 6-8-2? 6-8-2 becomes what？

3 桁をクリアできれば、次は 4 桁です。

● Great, that's right. Let's go to four digits. 3-5-2-9 becomes what?

★ できなかった時のフォローも忘れずに！

● Don't feel bad.

● Don't worry.

● That's okay. I know it's a really difficult question.

7．それでは先ほど私が言った、3つの言葉を教えてください。

● Can you please tell me the three words I told you a few minutes ago?

I said three words a few minutes ago, didn't I?

言えた場合：Excellent！Wonderful！

言えなかった場合：助け舟として、Let me give you a hint. Shall I give you a hint? The first one was … a kind of flower…? The second one was … a kind of animal? The third one was … a kind of vehicle…?

8．5つの物品を覚えてください

「さて、これから5つのものをお見せします。順番は問いません。この箱の中に何が入っていたかをよく覚えてください。これはなんですか？　そうですね」と物品の名前を確認しながら、運動性失語や失認、意味性失語の鑑別を行ってください。そして私は、しばしば一緒に来たご家族も巻き込んで検査します。

● Now, I'll show you five items. Don't worry about the order. Just remember what's inside the box.

● So, what's this? → "It's a pen." → That's right.

と5つの物品の名前を確認する。

（そしてクリニックに患者さんを連れてきたのが娘さんだった場合……）

I bet your daughter is trying to keep up with you in her mind！と冗談めかしてみるのはどうでしょうか？

● I'm going to close the box now.（さぁ 箱を閉めますよ〜）

9. 片手でOK、片手できつねを作ってください（左右失認や視空間失認のチェック）

[立体形態の変換]

例えば、「右手で【OK】みたいな形を作ってください。」と言い、左右がわかるか？ また見た形を作れるか？（自分の手で再現できるか？）という二つの質問を同時に理解できるかどうか診ます。そして「今度は左手で【きつね】みたいな形を作ってください」と言います。その左右の形をいっせいのせで変換してもらいます。

● Please make this shape with your right hand. ⇐ OK 型

● Next, please make shape like this with your left hand. ⇐ きつね型

もう、like this が炸裂します！

● After I count to three, please switch the shapes to the other hands. One - two - three !

—— それでは 1・2・3 でいきますよ！

OK 型

きつね型

これは結構難しいので、がっくりさせないように注意が必要です。

できた時：Great! Good! That's correct. Very nice. Wonderful! Excellent !

できなかった時：That's close. Don't worry. It's a very difficult task. That's not bad.

[Barre's Sign]

● Stretch your arms forward like this, close your eyes and hold this position for 10 seconds.

——こんな風に腕を出して目を閉じて10秒保ってください。(Dr. が見本を呈示する)

または

● Can you extend your arms with palms facing the ceiling and hold them there for 10 seconds?

　　── 手掌を天井に向けてそのまま10秒頑張ってください。

● I'll start to count now.　Here we go.

　1 - 2 - 3 - ……. 10. OK. Please open your eyes. Thank you.

★ 次のtestに移るとき：Let's move on to the next test.

[手指失認]

● Spread your fingers like this.

　　── 手の指と指を広げてください。

● Close your eyes, and when I touch one of your fingers, please tell me which it is.

　　── 目を閉じて、私がどの指に触ったか教えてください。

● Keep your eyes closed.

　　── 目は閉じたままですよ〜。

● Which one is it？

　OK. Which is this?

　OK, and how about this one?

　OK, thank you.

手の指を広げてもらい、目を
つぶったまま、どの指に触っ
たか答えてもらう問いです。

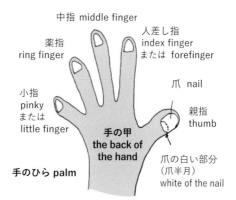

中指 middle finger

人差し指 index finger または forefinger

薬指 ring finger

爪 nail

小指 pinky または little finger

親指 thumb

手の甲 the back of the hand

爪の白い部分（爪半月）white of the nail

手のひら palm

10. 野菜の名前を10個言ってください

● Please tell me the names of 10 vegetables. Anything is OK. Please start now.（please go ahead.）

11. それではさっき箱にしまった5つの物品を教えてください

● Now, please tell me the five items I showed you in the box. Do you remember what was in it?

もし患者さんが何も言えない、もしくはその検査を忘れている、と考えられるとき、こんなふうに言うのはどうでしょう？
If your patient can't remember any of the objects, you might be able to say something like this.

● Let's take a look.
　── ちょっと見てみましょうか（と、箱を開けてみる）。
● Was this really here before?
　── これ、ここにありましたっけ（と、見た記憶が残っているか確認する）。
● Have you seen this before?
　── これ、ご覧になりましたか？
そして
● This is the end of this exam. Thank you. Good job.
　── これで一通りの検査は終了です。ありがとうございました。お疲れさまでした。

いかがでしたか。うまく、HDS-R できましたか。

診察が終わり、声をかけてあげるとすれば……

　患者さんが診察室から出ていくとき、どのように声をかけていますか？

　日本語では、「どうぞお大事になさってくださいね」とか「陰ながら応援していますからね～！！」とか「頑張っていきましょうね。必ずよくなりますから」とか「もし何かあったら相談してくださいね」など、言っています。患者さんが治療を継続していきたくなる工夫は必要だと思います。

　普通の英語診察の教科書には、

Please take care of yourself.

Take it easy.

と書いてありますが、Bret先生に、どう言われるのがいいですか？ と聞いてみました。すると Bret先生は「きちんと丁寧に患者さんの名前を呼ぶのが大切！」とおっしゃいました。なるほど！ と思いました。

Take care of yourself, Mr. Vector.

I'm sure you will be feeling better soon.

Don't worry, Mr. Vector. You will get better soon.

If you have any questions, please don't hesitate to ask.

If something comes up, please feel free to contact me during our office hours.

　そして日本語での日常診療にも必要と思いますが、次の来院を明確にしましょう。

See you again on June 12th, Mr. Vector.

または

Please come again in two weeks, Mr. Vector.

などでしょうか。 精神科は特に、確実によくなるまで見届けたい科ですからね。

次の第二章では
診断、処方決定、薬の説明をします。

それぞれ
各論を参考にしてください。
精神療法も少し書かれています。

そして第三章では、
日々の診療に役立つ小話を
載せています。

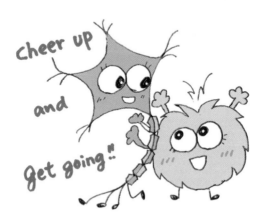

各 論

DETAILS

6つの症例について

ここでは架空の新患症例を通して、いろんな質問の仕方、薬の注意の仕方、疾患に対する患者さんへの教育的助言について学んでいきましょう。

　ここに出てくるのは、皆さんが日常臨床でよく遭遇するであろう仮想の患者さんです。6 例考えてみましたので、想像しながらお読みください。

　精神科という科は、他の科と趣を異にしています。
　たいてい他の科では、患者さんは何かの自覚症状があって診療所・病院に訪れるわけですが、精神科では多くの患者さんが症状を認識しないので、しばしば本人を説得して医療機関に連れていくのが大変です。

　ですから、せっかく来てくれた患者さんたちを傷つけることなく、診断に必要で大切な情報を得ることが重要と考えます。

　In other medical departments, patients usually come to the hospital or clinic voluntarily when they feel something wrong. However, within psychiatry, most patients do not recognize their symptoms and it is sometimes very hard to persuade them to come to a medical institution.
　Therefore, the most important thing is to get crucial diagnostic information without wounding the patient's pride.

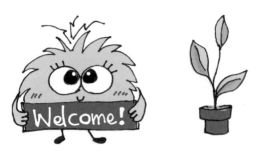

CASE 1

Mrs. Margaret Green A Ninety-year-old Woman Showing Signs of Cognitive Disorder

～認知症が疑われる老婦人～

マーガレット・グリーンさんは娘さんと二人暮らしです。娘さんは仕事が忙しく日中は独居です。高度な老人性難聴はありますが、年齢に比し日常生活動作はほぼ自立しています。ところが、最近心配なことが出てきました。

グリーンさんは物忘れと音楽性幻聴で困っています。今日は、グリーンさんの意に反して娘さんにクリニックへ連れてこられました。

Mrs. Green has auditory hallucinations and forgetfulness. Her daughter brought her to the clinic against her will today. Because she didn't actually want to come herself, I want to be careful to show respect for her feelings.

だからこそ、こんなふうに迎え入れてあげたいと思います。

● Welcome to our clinic. I know it might have been a difficult decision to come today, but I am so grateful that you did, Mrs. Green. I really respect your courage.

――ようこそこのクリニックにいらっしゃいましたね。お気持ちとそぐわないことはわかっていますが、グリーンさんがいらしてくださり、よかったと思います。とても勇気があると思いますよ。

いざ、診断の時です。

HDS-Rや神経学的所見を取らせてもらい、できれば頭部MRIなど画像診断を確認したのち、まずは認知症のご本人に、「まだまだできることはたくさんあるのだから、現在のお力を維持していくのが大切です」と、こんなふうに言うのはどうでしょう？

● According to today's examinations, I'm afraid you might be suffering from a certain degree of memory loss, but it's not enough to worry about.

You can sleep, eat well and you have a wonderful smile. You can also walk, get dressed by yourself and even grow vegetables in your garden, Mrs. Green. I want to help you maintain your current abilities as long as possible.

高齢者の（特に聴覚障害、難聴がある場合）幻聴は臨床ではよくあることですが、認知症のご本人にとっては、現実見当識や理解力の低下なども相まって、すごく辛い一大事だと思います。そして不安や孤独な環境から起こることが多く、その環境調整も重要です。

● It's actually not so rare to hear songs or even voices. Because you said you didn't hear the songs while we were talking today, I think you should try to talk with others more often. For example, why don't you take part in what we call "Day service" activities. You can apply for them, using the long term care insurance system (Kaigo-hoken) in Japan. Talking to people other than your family members will help keep your brain active. I really recommend talking with others as much as possible, because it can protect you from the memory loss that you worry about.

――（高齢者の）音楽性幻聴は、決して珍しくなく、結構多くの方が経験します。今日診察室でお話しているときは音楽が聞こえていなかった、とおっしゃったでしょ？ ですから、例えば介護保険制度を利用してデイサービスなどに参加してみるのはいかがでしょうか。ご家族以外の方とお話しすることで、脳は活性化されます。すごくおすすめです。そうすることで、心配していらっしゃる物忘れも防ぐことができますよ。

とお話ししてみることが多いです。結構「そうね」と同意してくださる方は多いですが、いずれ忘却のかなた……の場合も。それでも元気づける方法で説得していきましょう。

　私の場合、初診ではまず患者さんご本人の診察をして、そしてご家族のお話を聞くようにしています。そのため、患者さんにひと言断ることが必要です。

● Next, I'd like to talk to your daughter about her observations of your condition at home. Could you wait here for minutes?

ご家族へ質問します。

● When did you first notice something was wrong (or unusual) with your mother?
　——いつごろからお母様の変化に気づいていらっしゃいましたか？

> この時、something strange とか something abnormal とお聞きするのはネガティブなイメージらしいので避けたほうがいいみたいです。

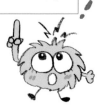

● What is the most serious problem for your family?
　——何について一番困っていますか？
● How does she spend her time at home?
　——家でどのようにお過ごしですか？

【排泄】
これは患者さんの前で質問するのにはとてもデリケートな問題ですが、聞かないわけにはいきません。「トイレは間に合っていますか？」
● Does she usually get to the restroom in time?
● Has she ever wet her pants or bed?

これは子供などにも使える婉曲表現だそうです。

【歩行】

● Does she go for walks alone or with someone from your family?

——おひとりで出かけられますか？ それとも外出は家族と一緒ですか？

● Has she ever fallen down?

——転んでないですか？

● Has she fallen down within the last three months?

——この3か月ぐらいで転んだこと、ありましたか？

【患者さんの今後について】

● What do you think about her situation?

What kind of care do you think would be best for your mother in the future?

——現状をどのようにお考えですか？

将来的にはどんな介護を想定されていますか？

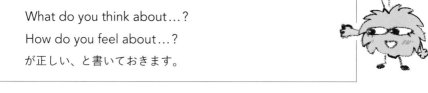

＊中学生のようで恐縮ですが……私自身の混乱をなくすために

What do you think about…?

How do you feel about…?

が正しい、と書いておきます。

● My initial impression, based on today's examination, is that she suffers from vascular dementia. In order to maintain her current abilities, it will be necessary to carefully treat her diabetes and hypertension as well.

—— 今日の診察を踏まえ、初診時診断としては、血管性認知症と考えられます。

そして糖尿病と高血圧をいい状態に保つことが認知症を進めないために大切です。

● If she has a Japanese health insurance card, she can use the welfare system for elderly people. To use the system she has to apply at a public office (or local government office).

　——日本での健康保険証をお持ちであれば、高齢者向けの制度があります。それを使うには、役所に届け出る必要があります。

そして最後に患者さんへ。

● We are going to do everything we can to let you stay active and positive!

　——まだまだお元気で過ごせるように支援していきますので、安心していてください。

● It is important and nice to enjoy healthy meals, but please don't eat too much, and don't forget to take your anti-hypertension medication every day, Mrs. Green. Regular exercise will also be good for you.

　——お食事が楽しいのはよいことなのですが、食べ過ぎないようにお願いしますね。そして血圧のお薬は忘れないようにしてくださいね、グリーンさん。適度な運動もいいですよ。

● Please come back again in two weeks.

　——また2週間後にいらしてください。

グリーンさん、少し元気になってくれたでしょうか？

Mr. Tom Vector A 36-year-old Employee of an IT Company Married with a One-year-old Child

~胃痛に悩む壮年男性~

トム・ベクターさんはとても忙しいIT企業にお勤めの男性です。最近胃のあたりが痛むことを心配して近医の内科にかかり、胃カメラ検査もしましたが、内科的には異常なしとして、精神科受診をすすめられました。

One month ago, Mr. Vector had a stomachache. He went to a family clinic, and the physician found nothing abnormal physically. Nevertheless, the pain remained for a long time and he saw the physician again. Mr. Vector was then advised that he should see a psychiatrist or visit a mental clinic. Blood and gastro-endoscopic examinations showed results within normal limits.

そして質問用紙を確認した後……

● Do you feel pain in your stomach today? Can you show me exactly where you feel it?
　──今も痛みは続いていますか？ どのあたりですか？

● When did it start? Is it constant or intermittent? Did it begin gradually or suddenly?
　──それはいつ始まりましたか？ 持続的ですか間欠的ですか？ 徐々に痛みが出てきますか？ それとも突発的に痛みますか？

● What kind of pain is it, sharp, dull, burning, stinging or tight?
　──痛みの性状は？ 鋭いような、鈍痛、焼けつくような、刺すような、締め付けられるような……どんな感じですか？

● How long does the pain continue? Seconds? Minutes? Hours?
　　── その痛みは何秒、何分、何時間ほど続きますか？

● How long does it usually last?
　　── たいてい、どのくらい痛みは続きますか？

● Does the area of pain move?"
　　── その痛みはあちこち動きますか？

● Does the pain occur before meals, during meals or after meals?
　　── 痛いのは食前、食べている最中、食後としたらいつですか？

● Does anything make it better or worse?
　　── その痛みは何かでよくなったり、悪くなったりしますか？

● Was there anything else associated with the pain, for example sweating or vomiting?
　　── 痛みとともに発汗や嘔吐などありますか？

● Do you have an appetite recently?
　　── 最近、お腹すいたって思いますか？

● Is your weight steady?
　　── 体重はお変わりありませんか？

● Do you have regular bowel movements?
　　── 便通はいかがですか？

少し踏み込んで聞いてみることにします。

● I'm afraid I have to ask you many personal questions.
　　── 少し個人的なことまでお聞きします。

● Have you had any particular trouble which causes you stress?
　　── ストレスと考えられるような何かはありましたか？

● Is there any event that you feel could have caused the stomachache?
　　── 胃が痛くなるくらいの出来事はありましたか？

● Have you had any trouble at home or at work?
　　── 家庭で、または職場で、お困りのことはありますか？

● How long do you work in a day?
　　── 一日何時間労働ですか？

そして、食欲・睡眠についてチェック！
（第1章　P17~18「精神的症状の所見として」を参考にしてください）

● Do you drink alcohol? How much do you drink in general? Every day?
　　── お酒類は、一日どのくらい摂られますか？（アルコールに問題がある方
　　は特にすごく控えめに申告されるので、正直にお話していただきましょう）

● Do you like spicy food? What kind of hot things do you like?
　　── 辛い物は召し上がりますか？ どんな感じですか？

● Do you like coffee or tea? How much coffee do you drink every day?
　　── コーヒーや紅茶などお好きですか？ どのくらい飲みますか？

● Do you like carbonated drinks? Do you care for cold drinks?
　── 炭酸飲料はいかがですか？冷たい飲み物はお好きですか？

● Do you have any other symptoms, including headaches, shoulder pain, palpitations, dizziness, vertigo or diarrhea?
　── ほかに気になる症状はありますか？例えば頭痛・肩こり・動悸・めまい感・回転性めまい・下痢などですが。

● Have you ever felt sick during a blood sampling?
　── 採血の時に気持ち悪くなったことはありますか？

● Are you allergic to alcohol wipes?
　── アルコール消毒のアレルギーはありませんか？

　これらの根掘り葉掘りの質問をし、身体的・神経学的所見を取りましたが、それでも体の緊張が強いぐらいで異常なしでした。「やはり、ストレスを感じやすい方で、前医での内科的に異常なしを踏まえ、精神科的アプローチが必要そう」と初診時診断をしたとします。

● My initial impression, based on what we have done today, is that you suffer from somato-form-disorder (or stress related disorders). Just as every coin has two sides, the body and mind are linked together. So, if it is difficult to cure your pain from a physical side, it is a good idea to try to approach the pain from a psychiatric perspective. In a way you are lucky because the tests done by Dr. XXX（前医）show that you have no physical illness. Because we can be confident in that, we can concentrate your treatment from the psychiatric side. You have no need to blame yourself. Mental illness doesn't reflect on your character or intelligence at all. As a first step, we will try some medications to help with your energy levels and ease your stomachache. Then as the next step, we will talk about stress management, after you begin to feel better physically.

――今日いろいろとおうかがいして、初診時としては、身体化障害（ストレス関連性障害）と考えられます。コインにも裏と表があるように、体と心もつながっています。体の症状で内科的に難しければ、精神科的なほうから胃痛に対しアプローチするのもありだと思いますよ。ベクターさんの場合、内科的に問題がないことは前医からの検査でお墨付きなわけですから、喜んでいいことですよ。そうしたら精神科的な方法に集中できますから。ご自分を責める必要はありません。このタイプでは、精神疾患は性格が弱いというわけではありません。まずはエネルギーを貯め、痛みを和らげるために薬を処方します。そして、よくなってきたら、次のステップでストレスマネージメントの方法について話し合っていきましょう。

● In order to ease the pain, I'll give you two types of medication today, Mr. Vector. One is an anti-depressant and the other is a minor tranquilizer. You should take them before sleeping at night. They should also help with your insomnia since both of them might make you sleepy. The side effects of the anti-depressant might include constipation, nausea, dry mouth or sleepiness. Be careful regarding the timing when taking the drugs. Please avoid driving and dangerous work after taking them because this medicine will make you sleepy. If these medications are effective, your symptoms should disappear in about two weeks.

――ベクターさん、痛みを和らげるために、今日2種類の薬を差し上げます。ひとつは抗うつ剤でもうひとつは抗不安薬です。夜、就寝前に服用し

てください。両方とも眠気が生じますので、夜はよく眠れると思います。抗うつ剤の副作用は便秘・吐気・口喝・眠気です。お薬は使うと眠くなりますので、運転や危険な作業はお薬を飲んだ後にはやらないでください。お薬は効果があれば2週間で効いてくると思いますよ。

● However, please note that you should continue to take the medicines for at least three or four months even if you have no more stomachache. This is a very important point. Our brains are clumsy. It will take a little bit of time for your neurological system to repair its neurotransmitter condition. If you stop taking the medicines too early, the symptom might relapse. I really hope that you will get better and not have to visit us anymore. Do you have any questions?

　――ただし、症状が取れても、3～4か月はお薬を続けてくださいね。それ、とても大切なんです。我々の脳って、ぶきっちょ（不器用）なんですよ。神経伝達物質などの状態を整えるのに、時間がかかってしまうのです。早くにお薬を中断すると再発する心配があります。きちんとよくなってもらいたいのです。何かお聞きになりたいことはありますか。

● Take care of yourself, Mr. Vector. I'm sure you will be feeling better soon. See you again in two weeks. Can you make an appointment for your next visit on your way out? We don't have a pharmacy within the clinic but we will issue a prescription that you can take to any pharmacy you like. If you don't know where to go, we can show you some pharmacies.

　――どうぞお大事になさってくださいね、ベクターさん。早くよくなるといいですよね。また2週間後にいらしてください。次回の予約をお願いします。このクリニックでお薬をお渡しできないのですが、処方箋をお出しし

ますので、ご存じの薬局で薬をもらってください。もし薬局をご存じなければお教えいたしますよ。

Vectorさんも、生活習慣全般を見直して、健やかにお過ごしになれますように!

英語の勉強をしていて、あまりに進展がないためにがっかりすることは多々あります。もう、しゅんとして投げやりな気持ちになってしまいませんか? そんな時は……こんなふうに励まされるのはどうでしょう?

● What doesn't kill you makes you stronger!(哲学者ニーチェ)

● Where there's a will, there's a way.
（第16代アメリカ合衆国大統領リンカーン）

● There is nothing to fear but fear itself.
（第26代アメリカ合衆国大統領ルーズベルト）

Life is full of obstacles, but we can learn from those experiences and move on! There's always room for improvement.
ほら、元気出てきましたか?

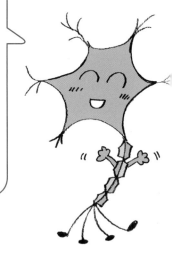

CASE 3

Mr. David Stingray A 70-year-old Man with Sleeping Problems

~不眠を訴える老紳士~

「寝床に入り、すぐに眠れないから睡眠薬が欲しい」とお手軽に考えて受診された 70 歳のデイビッド・スティングレーさん。さて、すぐにお薬……ではなく考え方や生活習慣を軌道修正してもらえるように上手に説得できるか？が問題です。

　クリニックでは、とてもよくいらっしゃいます。「つべこべ言わずに睡眠薬をよこせ！」という患者さん。

　精神科ではそうはいきません。初診では根掘り葉掘りおうかがいします。もちろん守秘義務は厳守いたします。

　Since retiring at 65, Mr. Stingray gradually began to suffer from insomnia. He has hypertension and hyperlipidaemia, neither of which is controlled well now. He is generally inactive in the daytime. After retiring, his daily alcohol consumption has increased.

　Mr. Stingray feels anxiety regarding "sleep". Such anxiety doesn't have a relationship to whether he can sleep well or not.

　Although most patients with insomnia are eager to get sleeping pills and take them instantly in order to fall asleep very quickly, the goal for them is to improve their QOL (quality of life), not just to sleep longer.

　65 歳で定年後、スティングレーさんはだんだん眠れなくなってきました。高血圧と高脂血症と言われていますが、コントロールは現在不良です。日中の活動性も少なく、定年を迎えてからはお酒の摂取量も増えています。

　とにもかくにも「眠り」への不安をもちですが、それは現実的によく眠れたかどうかとはあまり関係がありません。不眠を抱える多くの患者さんは、睡眠薬で「手っ取り早くすぐに眠りにつきたい」と考えがちなのですが、治療のゴールは生活の質の向上であって、「ただ早く長く眠れりゃいい」というわけではありません。

　Clearly, the most important thing for us as doctors is to persuade these patients to improve their insomnia by making positive lifestyle changes.

さて、うまく説得できるでしょうか？

　初診ですから、質問用紙を念入りにチェックし、神経学的所見を取り、内科に行っていればよし、行っていなければ採血をさせてもらいます。そのうえで、質問です。

● How many hours of sleep do you think is necessary for people of your age?
　ースティングレーさんぐらいのお年の方は、どのくらい睡眠時間が必要と思われますか？

　多くの不眠に悩む方は、8時間ばっちり寝ないとダメと思い込んでいる方が多いように思います。

● 6～7 hours of sleep is enough for elderly people, Mr. Stingray. Moreover, spending excessive time in bed may actually disturb the quality of your sleep at night.
　ー6～7時間で十分ですよ。それに、あまり長くお布団に入っていると睡眠の質が悪くなっちゃうんですよ。

● Do you feel sleepy during the daytime?
　ーお昼間の眠気はありますか？

　「自分は不眠症！」と思い込んでいる方の中には、眠気を感じても、「夜眠れないと困るから」と必死で昼間に起きていようとする方も多いですね。眠くなければあえて寝ることはありませんが、もし眠いのであれば……。

● You might feel anxious that if you sleep in the daytime, you won't be able to fall asleep at night. However, don't worry about that. It is okay to sleep up to one hour between one and three o'clock in the afternoon. Taking a nap for a short time doesn't disturb your sleep at night. In fact, it even helps avoid the risk of dementia, epidemiologically speaking.

――午後 1 時から 3 時の間で 1 時間以内寝るのはかまいませんよ。「お昼間に寝ちゃうと夜眠れなくなっちゃうんじゃないか」と心配なんですよね。心配いりません。疫学的には、むしろ昼間の短い睡眠は認知症のリスクを下げると考えられています。

● Do you try to get more sleep by going to bed earlier and earlier?

――もっと寝ようと思って、寝床に入るのがどんどんはやくなっていませんか？

● It is said that the longer you stay in bed without sleeping, the poorer the quality of your sleep will be. It's a vicious circle!

――寝床に入ったまま寝ないでいる時間が長いと睡眠の質を下げてしまうし、それこそが悪循環ですよ。

● Taking medicine (sleeping pills) is one way to improve insomnia, but it's not the first choice. I can't emphasize that enough. Taking sleeping pills is just a short time solution, not a cure. The goal is to improve your QOL(Quality of Life), not just to sleep longer. The effectiveness of sleeping pills varies from individual to individual. No one can predict their effectiveness before actually using it. I don't mean to scare you, but sleeping pills might cause delirium especially in elderly people. Usage of sleeping pills must be undertaken carefully by people like you.

——睡眠薬も一つの選択肢なのですが……一番にお薬！ではありません。大切なことを言いますよ。お薬を飲んで眠れたからって、本当に治ったことにはなりません。大事なのは、生活の質を向上させることで、ただ長く寝むれりゃいいわけではありません。睡眠薬の効果は個人差が大きいですし、ね。使ってみないとわからないのです。怖がらせるわけではないのですが、高齢の方はせん妄を起こすこともあります。だから大変注意が必要なのです。

● I don't recommend just taking sleeping pills without first trying to adjust your life rhythm, improve your sleep hygiene, control your hypertention and reduce your alcohol intake. Proper exercise would be good for your sleep, as well. It is also said, "Sleeping late and getting up early" condenses your sleep, and the quality will improve.

——だから、生活リズムを整えたり、睡眠の質を考えたり、血圧を安定させるのも大事です。それとお酒も控えましょう。ほどよい運動も睡眠にはとてもいいんですよ。また、『遅寝・早起き』も睡眠の質を上げると言われていますしね。

● Surprisingly, there are some people who believe that alcohol gives them good sleep, but the truth is completely the opposite. In fact, alcohol is a stimulant which wakes up the brain. Drinking too much causes loss of consciousness, but not good sleep. If you want to sleep well, you should reduce your alcohol intake. If you don't do that, I can't give you any sleeping pills.

——お酒を飲むとよく寝れると思っている方がおられますが、まるっきり逆なんですよ。びっくりでしょ。お酒は頭を起こす薬物なんですよ。お酒を飲んで意識を失うことはありますが、それは良質の睡眠とは言えないんですよ。ぐっすり寝たいとお思いならば、お酒は控えてください。そうできなければ、睡眠のお薬は差し上げられません。

これ、決め台詞です！！

● If alcohol were effective for the treatment of insomnia, all psychiatric clinics would be pubs!

　——もしお酒が不眠症の治療になるのなら、精神科の診療所はみーんな居酒屋になっちゃってますよ！

● There are several points to SHE (Sleep Hygiene Education). I'll give you a simple overview now.

❶ Make sure your sleeping room is dark and quiet.

　——寝室は暗く静かに。

❷ Turn off all TVs, computers, and smartphones.

　——テレビ、パソコン、スマートフォンの電源を切りましょう。

❸ Go to bed at the same time every night, even if you have a plan to get up early the next day.

　——明日に早起きする予定があっても、いつもと同じ時間に就寝しましょう。

❹ List in your mind three happy events that happened that day.

　——今日起こったいいことを３つ書き出してみるのもいいですね。

❺ Relax and smile.

　——リラックスして、笑顔笑顔 。

❻ Please don't mull over any negative events of the day in your bed.

　——お布団の上では、嫌なことはなるべく考えないように。

❼ Finally, get up at the same time every morning. Be sure to open the windows to let the morning light into your eyes, which helps to regulate your circadian rhythms.

──同じ時刻に起床して、窓をあけ、朝の光を目に取り込みましょう。そうすると生活リズムを整えることができます。

● Can you accept my advice and try these steps?

──できそうですか？

● Please try to do each of these things for two weeks, and I promise you will find your sleep improving naturally. From this first visit, I think there are many things that you can do to improve in your daily life, so I'm not going to give you sleeping pills today, Mr. Stingray. Again, take care of your hypertention, don't drink too much and follow the SHE protocols. Please come again in two weeks. Do you have any questions? Above all, please take care of yourself as kindly as you would someone you love. It is important to be kind to yourself.

──まず2週間、やってみてください。すごくよくなると思いますよ。日常生活での改善点がいくつもありそうなので、今日はお薬をお渡ししません。血圧のお薬忘れずに、お酒もほどほどに、そしてSHE（Sleep Hygiene Education）をやってみてくださいね。また2週間後にいらしてください。何かお聞きになりたいことはありますか。なんだかんだ言っても、自分を大切にしましょうね。

スティングレーさんはわかってくださったでしょうか？

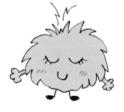

こんな言葉も素敵です。

An ounce of prevention is worth a pound of cure.
（１オンスの予防は１ポンドの治療の価値がある）

If alcohol were
effective for
the treatment of insomnia,
all psychiatric clinics
would be pubs!

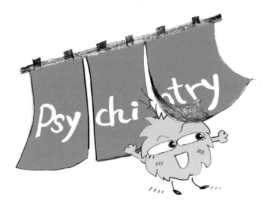

Sometimes a little good
advice is the best medicine!

CASE 4

Mrs. Monica Brown A 36-year-old Woman with Panic Attacks

〜パニック発作に悩む36歳女性〜

ブラウンさんは動悸と呼吸困難で、ここのところ3か月の間に救急車で2回運ばれていました。「気が狂ってしまうのではないか？」とか「死んでしまうのではないか？」と不安でした。心臓発作かと心配されたが、臨床検査では特に問題なし。それで精神科をすすめられたところです。ストレスを感じる出来事は特になかったと言います。アルコールやドラッグは否定。

During the past three months, Mrs. Brown was brought to the emergency room by ambulance twice due to palpitations and breathing difficulty. She said "I think I'm going crazy and I'm going to die." She was convinced that she was having a heart attack, but the results of physical and laboratory examinations were unremarkable. So, she was advised to go to a psychiatric clinic. There were no particular episodes that caused mental distress before the attacks. She denies drug use or excessive alcohol consumption.

そして質問用紙を確認した後……

● How long do the palpitations continue?
　　──動悸はどのくらい続きますか？

● Do you get nervous easily?
　　──緊張しやすいほうですか？

● Was there anything else associated with the palpitation and breathing difficulty?"
　　──動悸と呼吸困難のほかに何か症状はありますか？

● Have you had any stressful events recently which caused you stress?
　　──ストレスになるような心配なことはありませんでしたか？

● Do you like coffee or energy drinks?
　　──コーヒーやエナジードリンクは好きですか？

　質問用紙を含め、身体的・神経学的所見を行ったのち、やはりパニック障害のようだと伝えます。

● My initial impression, based on what we have done today, is that you suffer from panic disorder. This illness is not rare. In fact, about one person in a hundred has it.
　　──パニック障害だと考えられます。100人に1人ぐらいがなる、珍しいものではないです。

● Over the last ten years, we have seen many famous people confess that they suffer from panic disorder on TV shows, and I think that potentially there are even more.
　　──有名な人が自分はパニック障害だと告白しているのをこの10年でよくメディアで見るようになったが、潜在的にはもっといっぱいいるような疾患です。

● The autonomic nervous system is composed of the sympathetic and parasympathetic nervous systems. During panic attacks, the sympathetic nerves become too excited. You could say, it is like an emergency alarm malfunctioning. The alarm is ringing for no reason, which makes you scared, and your fear makes the alarm ring even more. It's a vicious circle. We can try to cut the circle by using anti-depressants. Panic disorder will definitely improve with proper treatment, although the amount of time needed to cure it depends on the individual. Choosing the kind and amount of anti-depressants to use is what we will focus on moving forward.

Let's start the first line of drugs today. If you have any trouble taking these medicines, please call me soon during our open hours. The main side effect you might experience from this medicine in the beginning is nausea. However, even if you don't experience this side effect, it doesn't mean the medicine isn't working. (The presence or absence of side effects has nothing to do with the medicine's effectiveness.) Nausea occurs in about 20% of patients who take it. If you vomit, please stop taking the medicine. Don't stop due to nausea alone. Since the side effect can last at most only four days, please try to endure it as much as possible. I'll give you a prescription for one week of stomach medication to help you. That is usually enough for most patients.

―― 自律神経の（交感神経と副交感神経がある中で）交感神経が過剰に緊張している状態です。例えて言うならば、非常ベルが誤作動を起こしているようなものです。ですから、理由なく非常ベルが鳴り、それがあなたを不安にさせ、ますますベルが鳴るという悪循環を起こします。この悪循環の輪を断ち切るのに、抗うつ剤が有効なことがあります。治療にかかる期間は人それぞれですが、パニック障害は、適切な治療で必ずよくなりますので、心配いりません。たくさんある抗うつ剤のうち、あなたに合う種類と量を選んでいくのが、あなたと私の共同作業です。

　まずは今日は、第一選択から差し上げますが、何か困った事があったら、遠慮なくおっしゃってください。この薬の一番よくある副作用は、飲み始めの吐き気です。副作用が出ないからといって、薬の効果がないわけではありません（副作用の有無と効果発現は関係がありません）。副作用は10

人に 2 人位と言われています。本当に吐いたら、やめてください。副作用は長くて 4 日なので、できれば乗り越えてください。飲み始めの一週間だけ、胃薬を一緒に差し上げます。それで大部分の患者さんは乗り越えられます。

● Although no abnormalities were found in your heart function, let me check for anemia and proper thyroid function because these could be the cause of your palpitations. And also, let me check your liver and kidney function before starting you on anti-depressants.

── 心臓には異常はなかったのですが、貧血と甲状腺はチェックさせてください。動悸の原因として最も考えられるからです。また、これから薬物療法を始めるにあたって、肝機能と腎機能もチェックさせてください。

● If your panic disorder is untreated, it could be dangerous because it might lead to secondary depression with risk of suicidal thoughts.

Have you ever thought you wanted to die?

Have you ever thought of a way to kill yourself on even prepared to do so?

I hope you never feel that way, but if you ever do-even a little-, please tell me as soon as possible before you do anything extreme.

Okay? Can you promise me not to kill yourself?

── パニック障害は、放っておくと二次性のうつ病を引き起こす危険があります。うつ病は自殺したくなってしまうこともあるので気をつけないといけません。

あなたは、死にたいという気持ちになったことはありますか？

そして、具体的な方法を考え、用意したことはありますか？

なければ結構です。少しでもあるようなら、いつでも連絡してください。いいですか？ 死なない約束、してくれますか？

● Please come back in two weeks. If you have any trouble with your medications, please call me during our office hours. If I am seeing another patient at the time you call me, I won't be able to talk with you, but I'll call you back as soon as I'm done, so please give us a telephone number where I can reach you easily. Since there is only one telephone in this clinic, we can't talk for a long time though. Anyways, please don't hesitate to ask me if you have a question.

―― 次回は2週間後にいらしてください。もしその間に、お薬のこととか心配があったら、いつでもお電話ください。私の診察中は電話に出られませんが、診察と診察の間にこちらから電話をしますので、受けられる電話番号を受付にお伝えください。クリニックの電話はひとつしかないので、長電話はできませんが。どうぞご遠慮なさらずに、ね。

ブラウンさん、きっと大丈夫ですよ！！

素敵な一言の紹介です。

◎ Nothing is impossible. The word itself says "I'm possible"!
 ― Audrey Hepburn

◎ Life is like riding a bicycle. To keep your balance, you must keep moving.
 ― Albert Einstein

Mrs. Caroline Stein with a Foreign Object in Her Throat

〜うつ状態で喉に異物感のある女性〜

52歳女性主婦。来日して1年のシュタインさん。徐々に食欲が減り、5kg体重減少と喉に何か詰まったような異物感を感じ始め、内科を受診しました。内視鏡検査・血液検査では特に異常はなく、精神科受診をすすめられました。

A 52-year-old housewife（homemaker）, it has been a year since Mrs. Stein came to Japan. She has gradually lost her appetite and 5kg in body weight. Because she also feels a ball like foreign object in her throat, she decided to see a physician. However, no abnormality was discovered by gastro-fiber scope or blood examination, so the physician said it was probably due to mental illness, and Mrs. Stein should see a psychiatrist.

　それでは……"What seems to be the problem?"とうかがう前に、シュタインさんはとても元気がなく不安で緊張している様子なので、このような事柄からお話を始めたほうがいいかもしれません。

● I'm afraid that I will have to ask you many personal questions, but you don't have to answer if you don't want to, Mrs. Stein. Rest assured that all information you share with me will be kept confidential. Even if your husband asked me about your condition, I couldn't answer without your consent. This room is even soundproof from the waiting room, so no one can hear us. This wall here is 18cm thick!
So, what seems to be the problem?
　──個人的なことをいろいろとおうかがいしなければなりませんが、シュタインさんが答えたくなければ、お答えにならなくて結構です。ただし、ここでお話されたことはどこにも出ませんのでご安心ください。万が一、ご主人があなたの状況を聞いてきても、あなたの同意なしにお話しできません。このお部屋は防音室なので、待合室からここでの会話を聞かれるこ

ともありません。この壁は 18cm の厚みがあるんですよ。

それでは、どうなさいましたか？

やはり、喉の異物感がお辛いようです。その症状についてお聞きします。

● First, tell me about the feeling in your throat.

Does it feel like an actual foreign object is in your throat?

Does the feeling continue all the time?

Does the feeling occur more strongly when you swallow foods?

Is the feeling accompanied by a burning sensation in your throat or does it feel like bitter or acidic indigestion?

── 初めに、喉の感じについて教えてください。

本当に喉に何かある感じですか？

常時その症状は続いていますか？

何か食べ物を飲み込んだ時、強く感じられますか？

喉の変な感じと一緒に焼けつくような痛みや、苦いものやすっぱいものがきたりしませんか？

女性で考慮しなければならないのは、月経やピルの使用、更年期障害などホルモンに関連した病態であると思います。

Hormone-related psychiatric symptoms are not uncommon- particularly in women, so it is important to ask about a women's menstrual cycle, use of contraceptive pills, and menopausal troubles.

そこで質問です。

● Do you have your menstrual period regularly?

── 生理の期間は規則的ですか？

● Have you ever felt discomfort before your period, including headaches, a stronger than usual appetite, sleepiness, constipation, diarrhea, irritability or depressive feelings?

——月経前に不快な症状を感じたことはありますか？ 例えば頭痛・過食になる・眠気・便秘・下痢・イライラする・落ち込んだ気持ちなど。

● Do you use the pill now? What is the reason for using it : for birth control or to regulate your menstrual cycle? Do you regularly see a gynecologist?

—— ピルは現在お使いですか？ 避妊のためですか？ それとも生理周期を安定させるためですか？ 婦人科に定期的に通われていますか？

● Do you have any trouble during your period? For example, abdominal pain or dizziness?

—— 生理中は腹痛やふらつきなどありますか？

● Have you ever experienced hypermenorrhea (heavy bleeding)?

—— 過多月経と思ったことはありますか？

● Do you feel menopausal trouble, such as hot flashes or sweating?

——更年期障害、例えばカーっと熱くなったり、汗が出たりなどありますか？

そして、人間関係についての質問です。

● Next, I'd like to ask you about your family.
Do you live with anyone？(Is there anybody who lives with you？)
Are you married？
Do you have any children？

Could you tell me about each child in order?

Are you experiencing any difficulties raising your children?

Do you have any trouble with your husband?

What does your husband say about your symptoms?

Are there any other people who you can talk to about your complaints?

——ご家族についてお聞きします。

今どなたかと一緒にお住まいですか？

ご結婚されていますか？

お子さんはいますか？

上のお子さんから順番にいくつか教えていただけますか？

子育て、大変と思ったことはありますか？

ご主人と何か問題はありますか？

ご主人はあなたの症状についてどうおっしゃっていますか？

困っていることを話せる方はいますか？

あら、大変。シュタインさんに対して、ご主人はこんなことを言うそうです。

● It's all in your mind. It's your imagination. You're just making it all up. There's no abnormal GF findings, so just think positively!

—— 気持ちの問題だよ。想像。自分で作り出しているんじゃないか。だって胃カメラも問題ないだろ。もっと前向きになれよ。

● Mrs. Stein, do you agree with his way of thinking?

What do you think about his ideas?

—— ご主人の意見、どう思われますか。

そして、聞きにくいことも……softly and directly……に質問します。

● Have you ever thought about suicide?

Do you ever wish you could run away from your problems?

—— 自殺とか、考えたことありますか？ どこかへ消えてしまいたいと思いますか？

それでは、うつ状態もあり、また内科的には問題なしと言われたが、確かに自分では症状を感じているシュタインさんへお話を続けていきましょう。

● Our bodies and minds are two sides of the same coin. Psychiatric treatment might work to improve your physical symptoms as well as your psychiatric symptoms. Believe it or not, symptom feeling a foreign object in your throat is a very common at any psychiatric department. If the symptom is truly due to a mental problem, it may be caused by a habit of not speaking your mind, or of keeping a secret against your will. It is said that this kind of dissatisfaction can cause you discomfort and make you feel like your throat is clogged.

—— 心と体はコインの裏と表みたいなものです。精神科的な治療が身体症状を改善することもあります。信じられないかもしれませんが、喉の異物感は精神科ではよくある症状なのです。その症状が気持ちからきているものであれば、それは言いたいことを言わないでいる習慣からきているかもしれません。その不満が喉の詰まりを作り出すこともあるみたいです。

● If you ever want to talk about anything, you can tell me about it-even topics you wouldn't discuss with other people. Expressing your opinion in words is very important.

—— 何かお話したいことがあったら、どうぞおっしゃってください。ちょっとほかの人に話せないようなことでも大丈夫です。思いを言葉にするのは大事なのですよ。

● No matter what others think about you, it is quite important for you to directly state your opinion. This is different from egotism. Even if you tell all your opinions to someone, he or she might not always understand the context. And of course, no one can understand you if you say nothing. People can seldom understand things before you tell them.

——誰がどう言おうと、思い切って自分の意見を言うのは大切なことと思います。それは自己中心的とは違います。言ったところで理解してもらえるとは限らないし、ましてや、言わなかったら何も伝わりません。

● Telling your opinion to someone consists of two stages.First, you must think in your mind about what you want to say, and then, only after this initial stage, can you tell it to others.During this first stage when you consider what to talk about and how to say it, you may even find the solution by yourself. Even if someone else can't give you good advice, you yourself can come up with a good idea on your own when you try to tell your opinion to me or somebody else. You shouldn't stay silent when you want to say something. You shouldn't hesitate to express yourself.

　And also, you shouldn't hesitate to say what you feel, because your opinions and your life itself matter.

——人に言いたいことを伝えるのって、2段階で成り立っています。いったん頭で何を言うか考えてから、次に初めて伝えられますよね。この初めに何を言おうか考えているときに自分の答えが見つかっちゃうかもしれません。私はいいアドバイスなんてできませんが、誰かに話そうとしたときに、いい案が浮かぶんですよ。黙ってちゃいけません。遠慮することはありません。

　あなたの人生そのものが意味のあるものなのですから、感じていることをはっきり言ったほうがいいですよ。

● Furthermore, even if everyone else in the world were your enemy, you yourself should be on your own side and be kind to yourself.

—— もっと言うと、もし自分以外の世界中の人が敵だとしても、自分は自分の味方で自分に優しくしてくださいね。

CASE 6

Mr. Bob Smith A 27-year-old Man is Brought to My Clinic by His Parents

～統合失調症疑いの男性～

ボブ・スミスさん27歳男性。10年以上自宅閉居の生活でした。今日は、ご両親がご本人を当院に連れてこられました。（一通り質問用紙に記入してもらい問診に入るとき、まず、ご本人の診察であることを明確にするため、ご本人にきちんとお聞きします）。

Mr. Bob Smith a 27-year-old man. He has been staying indoors for more than ten years. Today his parents brought him to the clinic.

● What seems to be the problem?

Did you want to come by yourself today, or did your parents bring you here against your will? Why do you think your parents wanted you to come? I know it must have been a difficult decision, but I'm so grateful that you came today, Mr. Smith.

—— 今日はどうされましたか？ ご自身で来院しようとされたのですか？ それともご両親が無理に連れてきたのですか？ どうしてご両親があなたをここに連れてきたと思われますか？ 大変だったと思いますが、よくいらっしゃったと思いますよ、スミスさん。

病感を探るため、質問を続けます。

● Can you sleep well at night, Mr. Smith?

Do you find yourself waking up several times in the night?

Do you ever have trouble falling back to sleep?

Do you wake up in the morning feeling very tired?

—— スミスさん、夜間はよく眠れますか？

何回も夜に起きたりしますか？ 一回起きるともう眠れなくなりませんか？ 朝起きた時、ぐったり疲れていませんか？

● Have you ever heard voices commanding you to do something?
　Can you describe these voices in more detail? Is it a male or a
　female voice?
　What did the voices say?
　Is this a common experience for you?
　(Have you ever experienced this kind of thing before?)
　Have you ever felt that someone was following you or watching
　you all the time?
　── 誰かの命令する声を聴いたことがありましたか？
　その声をもう少し詳しく説明できますか？　男性ですか？　女性ですか？
　声は何と言ったのですか？
　そういうこと、以前もありましたか？
　誰かにつけられたり、監視されていると感じたことはありますか？

　スミスさんはあまり自分では語ってくれないかもしれません。反応をひとつひ
とつ拾いながら……ですね。連れてこられたご両親にも話を聞きましょう。

● Mr. Smith, may I ask your parents a few questions, too?
　ースミスさん、ご両親にもお話を聞いてもいいですか？

● What seems to be the trouble with your son?
　How long have his symptoms continued?
　Is there anything else out of the ordinary you have noticed about him?
　Have you ever seen your son talking or laughing with someone you
　couldn't see?
　Does he often talk to himself?
　Has he ever been scared of something and you couldn't understand
　why? (Have you ever wondered why he was acting frightened?)

Has he changed from his previous self?

(Has his personality changed from what it used to be?)

── 息子さんについていかがですか？

どのくらいその症状が続いていますか？

何か普通と違うと気が付いたことはほかにありますか？

誰もいないのに息子さんが話していたり笑っていることはありましたか？

息子さん、独り言はよくありますか？

何かどうしてかわからないのに怖がっていたことはありますか？

昔の息子さんと変わったと思いますか？

● Does he have his meals with the family, or does he want to eat alone?

Does he regularly take a bath or shower?

Does he talk with both of you?

Does he spend time with anyone else?

Please tell me as much as you can about his lifestyle.

── 息子さんはご家族と食事をしますか？ それとも一人で食事しますか？

定期的に風呂とかシャワーで清潔を保てていますか？

お父様お母様と、息子さんはお話しされていますか？

どなたかほかの人と会ったりしていますか？

ほかに息子さんについて何かあったら教えてください。

Questions About Family History:

● Has anyone in your close or extended family ever had a psychiatric disease?

── ご親戚の中で精神科的病気であった人はいらっしゃいますか？

Questions About the Patient's Childhood

(including educational history) :

患者さんの発達・成長過程についての質問事項

● Did he have any health or social problems in kindergarten?
（幼稚園）

● How about during in elementary school, junior-high or high school?
（小・中・高校）

● What about college / university?
（大学）

In addition, the examining psychiatrists should carefully observe the patient's appearance, behavior, psychomotor activity, and attitude regarding the examiner. After performing physical examinations to rule out any other diagnosis, I would tell the patient and his parents as follows.

精神科医は患者さんの外観、ふるまい、精神運動性活動、治療者に対する態度などに注意を払いますよね。身体所見で鑑別診断をした後、こんな風に患者さんにお伝えします。

● Mr. Smith, I think there is a possibility you might have schizophrenia, although I'm not certain yet. It will take six months to confirm whether this diagnosis is correct or not. However, we should start treatment for your illness today. Once again, I think it would be in your best interests to start treatment as soon as possible from today.
—— スミスさん、おそらくは統合失調症と思われます。きちんと診断がつくまでは6か月かかりますけどね。それでも今日から治療を始めましょう。

● Generally speaking, schizophrenia is considered to be one of the most severe mental illnesses. However, it's not actually that rare. It is found in about 1% of the population. What is the cause of this illness? Various theories exist, but the most likely one is that schizophrenia is caused by a dopamine imbalance. Specifically, schizophrenia is thought to be caused by an excess of dopamine activity. By the way, do you know about neurotransmitters?

Neurotransmitters are chemicals that transmit signals from one neuron to another neuron. They are essential to the function of neural systems, so it is very important to maintain the balance of neurotransmitters.

Antipsychotic drugs can help to reduce dopamine activity, so with proper and suitable medication, your thoughts will become more orderly and clear. The medication helps to regain good neurotransmitter function. Therefore, you must continue to take the medication for a while. Please don't stop taking the antipsychotic drugs even if your symptoms disappear.

I really can't emphasize this enough!

── 一般的に、統合失調症は重い病気と思われがちですが、決して珍しい病気ではないんです。およそ１００人にひとり発病します。それでは原因はなんでしょうか？ 諸説ありますが、ドーパミンの不調により起こると言われています。ドーパミンがどばーっと出すぎてしまうんですね。ちなみに神経伝達物質ってご存じですか。神経脂肪から神経細胞へ情報を伝達する化学物質のことです。そのバランスを保つことがとても重要なのです。

お薬は出過ぎたドーパミンを減らす働きがあります。ですので適切な薬であなたの頭の中がもっとすっきりすると思いますよ。薬で神経伝達物質のいい状態を取り戻せると思います。ですので、しばらくお薬を続けてくださいね。症状が治まってもすぐにお薬をやめたりしないでくださいね！

すごく大事なことですからね！

● Antipsychotic drugs effect people in different ways, so if you have any side effects that make you feel uncomfortable, please tell me as soon as possible. Even so, antipsychotic drugs have improved dramatically in recent years, so they will surely help a lot. It generally takes three or four weeks for the effects of antipsychotic drugs to be felt.

── 精神のお薬は個人差が大きいですから、何か副作用かな、と思ったらすぐ教えてくださいね。精神科のお薬は最近とても開発が進んでいるので、結構いいですよ。おおよそ3〜4週間で効果を実感できると思いますよ。

● Please come back in two weeks.
We will help you get better little by little, Mr. Smith.
──スミスさん、次回2週間後に来院してください。少しずつよくなるようにと思っています。

スミスさん、次回少しよくなって来院してくれたら嬉しいな、と思います。

2回目に来た時……

● Hello, Mr. Smith. How have you been?
──いかがでしたか。

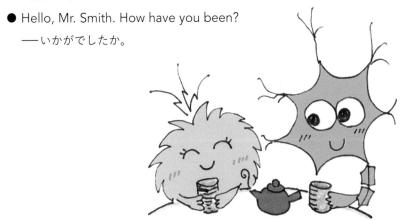

おまけのTerminology

auditory hallucination	幻聴
blocking of thought	思考途絶
catatonia	緊張病
delusion of persecution	被害妄想
delusion of reference	関係妄想
insight into disease	病識
loosing of association	連合弛緩
monologue	独語
thought of broadcasting	考想伝播
thought of hearing	考想化声
thought of insertion	考想吹入
thought of withdrawal	考想奪取

ちょっといい話

HANDY HINTS

~ Sometimes a little good advice
is the best medicine! ~

この章では、ちょっとした小ネタをお伝えしようと思います。

　臨床医は一人でたくさんの患者さんを受け持っていますから、いろいろな患者さんに同じ話をしていることに気が付きます。むしろ臨床医の能力は同じ話を何回も話せるか？にかかっているのではないかとさえ思います。

　そこで、こんなお話はいかがでしょうか。皆さんが患者さんに説明するとき、何かのお役に立てれば幸いです。

There are some short psychotherapy talks I often give patients in my clinic, and many patients tell me afterwards that they wish they had heard them much earlier. I hope these handy hints can help your patients overcome various difficulties in their lives.

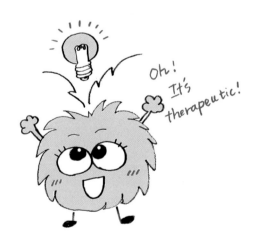

【不安の分別法のお話】

The Separation Method for Dealing with Anxiety

心配で心配でたまらない、という人いますよね。自分でもよくわかっちゃ
いるけどやめられない、みたいな人。そんな時、分別ごみよろしく、心配の
分別をおすすめしてみませんか。
　さて始めていきましょう。

I often talk to my patients as follows :

Everyone experiences anxiety.

In this clinic, too, there are a lot of patients with the symptoms of anxiety. Some have pathological anxiety which must be treated using evidence-based medicine just as any other mental illness. On the other hand, some patients simply worry too much, but within normal limits. If that describes you and you just want to get rid of excess anxiety, the following analogies and small bits of advice can help a lot.

First, if you are the type of person who worries too much, you should try to make the best of your personality as it is. Our personalities tend to be like coins with two sides. There is no bad character or good character. This means whether something is good or bad depends on one's perspective. For example, we can describe someone as "stubborn," but we could also say, he or she is "very strong-minded." The part of your character that you consider your weak point might actually be your strong point! Even if you think you are a negative-thinking person, such a negative part could have a positive influence. Here is one example.

When planning a big event like a picnic, positive-thinkers and negative-thinkers can have very different outcomes. The positive-thinker may just assume everything will go well, but the negative-thinker will be obsessed with the weather, traffic conditions, etc. The positive–thinker will probably be the life of the party, while the negative-thinker can steadily prepare for possible difficulties in detail. In reality, both can plan good events.

If you are an anxious person, please try to be a bit more confident. Have confidence that your unique contributions will be valuable in many situations. In this way you can capitalize on your strength.

That said, worrying about things too much can cause difficulties in your daily life. So, what should you do in that case?

I'd like to emphasize that there are three matters in life which we don't have to worry about. This leads to what I call "the separation method dealing with anxiety." If you can categorize your anxiety into one of these three issues, please try to stop thinking about it so much.

1. Don't worry about the past!

2. Don't worry about the distant future!

3. Don't worry what other people think about you!

Please make a decision today to reduce your anxiety with the following methods. Let me explain them in more detail.

1. Don't worry about the past!

As you know quite well, time will NOT come back no matter how much you worry about the past. This type of anxiety reduces your life energy. So how can you stop this kind of thinking? At such times, please remember President Kennedy.

What I mean by that is that it is no use saying such things as "If only President Kennedy had not been in Dallas that day, he would not have been killed." Worrying about your own past is the same as crying about him. If you think about the past again and again, please tell yourself to "Remember President Kennedy." This can be a mantra to help you stop thinking about the past.

2. Don't worry about the distant future!

Even with all your knowledge and life experience, you can't predict the weather of any day three years in the future. Nobody can know such a thing. If you can accept this fact so easily, why do you worry about your own future and things that may or may not happen three years from now? Such worrying is a waste of time.

If you worry about the future, you can stop thinking about it by remembering that you can't predict the weather in three years.

3. Don't worry what other people think about you!

Other people's minds belong to themselves. Nobody can dominate or control another person's mind. We must allow others the freedom to have their own opinions just as we are free in our own minds.

Please imagine that another person's thoughts are like their wallets. Naturally, because their wallets belong to them, we can't say anything like "Hey, I can see a dollar bill in your wallet. Use it quickly!" In truth, we can't even see inside their wallets! If you think this sounds strange or humorous, you are right! Other people's minds and attitudes are like the money in their wallets. You can't control other people's minds any more than you can control the money in their wallets.

If you find yourself worrying about someone's thoughts or attitudes, remember the dollar bill in your friend's wallet and it will help you stop thinking about it.

If what you are worrying about is not only this kind of trivial anxiety but something important that you should consider much more carefully in your life, you should think about the problem properly during the daytime, not at night (and especially not just before sleeping!).

If you tend to be a negative-thinker, it's not all bad because you can predict problems that could happen and prepare for them. Rather than worrying about future, please try to remember that all you can do is try your best to prepare for the future. Hope for the best, prepare for the worst. As the old saying goes, after rain comes fair weather.

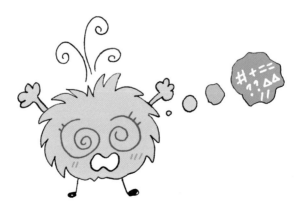

【休息のすすめ】

The Importance of Good Rest

　生き物にとって、休息はあらゆる場面で大切です。しかし人間は、勤勉さや向上心、競争心、しなければならない精神で休息がおろそかになってしまうことがあります。日々の臨床の中でも、本当はむしろ「寝るのも仕事だ！」と考えてほしい方、たくさんいます。
　ここでは、英語で休息のすすめをどう伝えるかを記したいと思います。

Again, I often talk to my patients as follows :

　When you feel tired, what do you do?
　It is crucial to take a rest when we are tired. It's not good to tell yourself that you are weak for resting. I don't recommend drinking energy drinks with excessive caffeine or alcoholic drinks in order to work harder during the day. We don't need superficial health. Please be kind and honest to yourself. Because humans are animals, it is impossible for us to continue working without rest like robots. It is necessary to get proper rest when needed. So, what is the best way to relax?
　I'd like to explain the way to get good rest, so you can learn how to take care of yourself.
　In fact, there are two types of rest. One is called passive rest, and the other is called active rest. Passive rest takes place when you lie down on a bed and relax. This type of rest is very important for the

treatment of all physical and mental diseases. Making your body horizontal helps reduce your blood pressure and the stress on your heart. (Your heart feels easier because it doesn't have to pump blood against gravity to your whole body.) Also, your internal organ blood flow may be increased in this posture. You can relax all your standing muscles as well. Please imagine that you have lain down in a comfortable position on the ground. You don't have to fall asleep. Just relax and take a rest on your bed. This is the first stage of good rest.

However, on the contrary, it is not good for your muscles or bones to lie still for a long time. (You have probably seen on TV shows that astronauts do exercises in space, otherwise they might get osteoporosis: a severe decrease in bone mass and density.) Stress from gravity is needed to maintain bone strength.

After this passive rest, and when you regain energy to stand up, you can advance to the next step: which is active rest. You can take a walk and feel comfortable in the gentle wind, play your favorite sports or even enjoy hiking. Active rest means feeling refreshed by using and moving your body within a comfortable range. Please don't overdo it.

When I talk about this idea, many people ask me "How can I know which type of rest I need at a given time?" The simple answer is that if you feel something would be impossible to do and you can't get up to do it, you are still in the earlier stage and you need to take passive rest. However, if you make up your mind about something, please don't hesitate to give active rest a try. This is a crucial point. You may now be in a stage of active rest. Active rest will help you relax more.

I hope you will rest effectively according to your needs, because I'm sure it will help you enjoy your life more fully. Someone can always cover your shift at work, but no one can replace YOU.

Counting the number of carp in a pond! ~ A Visualization Exercise

何かに迷ったとき、どうしますか？ という問題です。悩んでいても始まりません。どう解決につなげられるか？ が大切なのだと思います。

As a human being, there are many things to worry about in life. How do you deal with your problems? When we face something that makes us angry, sad or disappointed, we might think about it over and over. We might fall into confusion and begin to think in circles. Even if we decide to stop thinking about it, we might notice ourselves starting again. It can be hard when we can't find an exit from this endless loop.

Within psychiatry, we have an effective method to solve this type of problem. This is often described by the phrase "counting carp in a pond." Because carp in a pond swim freely, it's almost impossible for us to count them. Nevertheless, if you had to count them, how would you do it?

It would be impossible to count the carp as they swam quickly in all directions in the pond. Let me tell you the best way. The surest way is to prepare a new tank beside the pond and put the carp from the pond into the new tank one by one. Then you can count them easily. You no longer need to struggle at finding the carp within the unclear water of the pond.

Using this simple method, you can also make a list of your worries.

One by one, you can remove each problem from your brain.

Visualization of all the problems in your mind is just like "the counting of carp in the pond."

How can you do it practically?

1. If you have any anxiety or troubles, you should write each one down in a notebook, giving each one a specific label.

2. Make it clear to yourself when each one began, as well as in what situation you first noticed the thought and how it affected you.

The most important thing is to actually write them down by hand in a notebook, not only think about them in your brain. This allows you to see them objectively clearly. This is how we move each "carp" from the pond to the new water tank. Now you can visualize how many there are as well as their characteristics. You can grasp the crux of each issue this way. At the same time, you might also realize who you could go for advice.

3. If you are puzzled by two choices, I recommend you make a four-box table like this.

	Plan A	Plan B
Merits (Pros)	(I) ~~ ~~	(III) ~ ~~
Demerits (Cons)	(II) ~~ ~~	(IV) ~ ~~

Regarding Plan A, you should itemize as many of its merits as possible in (I), and demerits in (II) as many as possible. Regarding Plan B, you should itemize its merits in (III), and demerits in (IV) as many as you can consider. For example, if you are wondering whether to start a new job (plan A) or not (plan B), in (I) you could write: "I could enjoy my work more," "I could earn more money," and so on. In (II) "New stress will appear, other troubles might arise, and I would have to quit my current job…" In (III) "I could continue this stable life," "I know my colleagues well," and so on." In (IV) "If I lose this opportunity, I might regret it afterward," or "I'll be still dissatisfied with my current job."

After you fill in the blanks, you can easily compare each side to decide which the better course of action is.

What do you think about this method? By using it, you can be your own counselor because you've written down your problems and examined them.

Moreover, if a dear friend asked you for advice about the same problem, how would you answer them? I'm sure you would do your best to give good counsel. In this way your answer to your "friend" must be the best solution to your own problem.

I really recommend this visualizing exercise method in order to analyze your worries objectively. It may seem very simple, but it is much more effective than you expect. If you learn how to count up the carp in a pond, you will feel happier, and see your bright future more clearly. Never give up!

【 ハリネズミのジレンマ 】

The Hedgehog's Dilemma

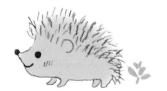

かわいいけれどトゲトゲのハリネズミさんたち。自然にはいろいろな生きるための工夫がいっぱいです。人間関係に悩んでいる方へのヒントがあります。

People tend to be very similar. Most people stumble at the same places.

Even though this is an old story, it's still fresh and helpful. Whenever I give this analogy in my clinic, my patients say "Oh, I see. I completely understand my situation from this story. Thank you, Doctor."

Hedgehogs are very cute mammals with sharp quills on their backs and the left and right sides of their bodies. During cold weather they try to get close to one another to share their body temperature. But, ouch!! It hurts! If they want to move closer together, they can't avoid hurting one another with their sharp quills. However, once they are separated, they feel cold again, so they approach each other once again. As you can already predict, they eventually hurt one another again. The hedgehogs don't want to be cold and lonely, but they hate to feel pain. After several attempts they find the optimal distance to be both safe and warm, and they all look very happy.

Arthur Schopenhauer made this story and Sigmund Freud used it to describe the proper distance for human relationships.

It is a good story.

I like it very much.

Life can be hard on occasion. Life has its ups and downs. If a relationship is too close, the people in it can sometimes hurt one another. However, if the relationship is too distant, they might feel lonely and isolated. A proper distance, providing warmth without pain, needs to be found.

At my clinic, I often talk to patients about their parent-child relationships (but I rarely discuss romantic relationships). There are a lot of people who struggle with their parent-child relationships, especially in the case of elderly parents and middle-aged children. The children want to care for their parents, but talk to them too frankly, which can naturally lead to quarreling. Even so, if the parents and children put too much distance between one another, they eventually start to worry about each another. Once again they approach, and once again they begin quarreling. Finally, disappointed with the tough situation, they come to talk to me about it. It is difficult to control these contradictory feelings.

As the cycle continues, my patients may be relieved and feel calm when they notice that they are experiencing the Hedgehog's dilemma. Like little hedgehogs many people fall into this pattern. With training, my patients realize how important proper distance is, and try to improve their relationship with their parents.

Human relationships seem to be based on trial and error. Please don't be afraid of making mistakes. With knowledge, we can move forward one step at a time. If hedgehogs can do it, so can we! I like to think so anyway.

In fact, in order to share their warmth, real hedgehogs often put together their cheeks, which only have small quills. This is also an impressive sign of ingenuity. Not to mention, very cute!!

If you are going through tough times, you are not alone.

Please try to smile and make the best of your relationship.

Above all, remember to breathe OUT calmly

　精神科では自律神経の中でも交感神経が過剰に興奮しているのではない
か、と思われる緊張の強い人が多くみられます。そんな中で、ふつうは意志
の力で動かせない自律神経のなかでも、リラックスにつながっている副交感
神経を自在にコントロールできたら、どんなに楽に過ごせるだろうな、と思
えることがあります。そんな方法のひとつを紹介できたら嬉しいです。物事
のやり方を伝えるって大変難しい技のひとつなのですけどね。

Have you ever seen a stray cat ruffle its fur when it meets a dog being walked on a leash? This behavior of the cat is evidence that its symptomatic nervous system is working.

As the cat breathed IN deeply, it likely had palpitations as its heart beat faster. Furthermore, its palms began sweat so as not to slip during a fight. Its pupils dilated, and its peripheral blood vessels contracted so as not to bleed easily during the fight. These are all instinctual reactions caused by the symptomatic nervous system to prepare the animal to fight.

The autonomic nervous system is the part of the nervous system that controls and regulates our internal organs without conscious input.

The autonomic nervous system is comprised of two antagonistic sets of nerves, the sympathetic and parasympathetic nervous systems. These two systems are basically antagonistic but also cooperate in order to regulate animal body functions. The sympathetic nervous system is effective for fighting. On the other hand, the parasympathetic nervous system is needed for relaxation. The sympathetic nervous system can be compared to a car accelerator, and the parasympathetic nervous system can be compared to a car brake.

Even while we are sleeping, both autonomic nervous systems are working constantly and seamlessly. The heart is beating, and each internal organ does its own work. Breathing in and out is accomplished by the cooperation of several muscles. The autonomic nervous system takes care of our whole bodies.

In addition, like that stray cat which I mentioned, the autonomic nervous system is often influenced by mental stress. It plays a direct role in our physical responses to stress. In fact, the central nervous system responds automatically to emergency situations or acute stress.

On the other hand, is there anything we can do to limit the effects of our autonomic nervous system's stress response? Yes, there is! In fact, there is one way to control the autonomic nervous system at will.

In general, it is impossible to move our intestines or to make our heart beat faster or slower at will. It is said that some great yoga masters can do it, but normally we are not able to do that kind of thing.

However, among the functions of the autonomic nervous system, it is only our beathing that we can control our system by ourselves. Breathing is usually an involuntary action, but we can also control our breathing by ourselves if we choose to. We can breathe deeply in and out and even hold our breath for a short time. For this reason, it can be possible to influence the autonomic nervous system through focused control of our breath.

The act of breathing IN is regulated by the symptomatic part of the autonomic nervous system, and breathing OUT is connected to the parasympathetic side which also controls relaxing in general.

When we take in a breath, our heart beats slightly faster, and when we let it out, our heart rate slows a little bit. Because the two nervous systems work alternatively, we are able to breathe in and out. (Our bodily functions are really amazing!) Though the parasympathetic nervous system usually regulates breathing out automatically, by exhaling on purpose, we can directly switch on the parasympathetic nervous system, which helps us relax at will. Doesn't that sound useful?

When we are tense for any reason, our bodies will naturally give priority to the sympathetic nervous system in order to deal with emergencies. However, if we actively choose to breathe out purposefully, we can shift control to our parasympathetic nervous system and begin to relax. This point is worth repeating. When we get nervous, our bodies naturally emphasize breathing in, but this is not always ideal because breathing in is connected to the sympathetic nerves which are meant to prime us for fight and will only increase our stress. In these moments, when you want to regain stability, please breathe OUT slowly to feel calm and relaxed.

Breathing is necessary for animal life and usually occurs without much thought. However, when you feel stress, try to breathe out deeply and slowly. Breathe OUT through your nose or mouth for ten seconds and IN through your nose for about five seconds. Though there are a lot of breathing techniques these days, just try this simple one if you feel nervous regarding an entrance examination for school, on the chair of a dental clinic, waiting in traffic jam, etc. Breathe out with your other muscles relaxed, too. This will help much more than you expect.

In addition, how many times have you heard the phrase: "to let out of a heavy sigh?" When we sigh with disappointment, frustration, annoyance, fatigue, or even if we sigh in relief, our sighs come out unintentionally. At that moment, the parasympathetic nervous system wants to help us relax by breathing out to release the stress. Therefore, even though a Japanese expression says, "Every time you sigh, happiness escapes," I think it is wrong. In fact, it's the exact opposite. Giving a sigh is good for your health. Please don't hesitate to sigh and let it switch on the parasympathetic nervous system for good relaxation.

Furthermore, in Japan jiggling your knee unconsciously is thought to be bad manners, but it is similar to chewing of gum by major league baseball players and can help you concentrate and relax. Whenever I see mothers stopping their children's legs from shaking, I always tell them that shaking legs is good for their children's mental health, even though it doesn't look good.

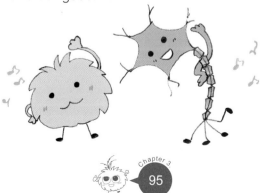

White Coat Syndrome

臨床医は同じような悩みをおもちの複数の患者さんに同じ話をしがちであると思います。そんな中で、とある一日に 3 人別々に同じ相談をされた経験をここでお伝えしましょう。

One day three separate patients each came to me with the same concern.

"Dr. Hiroko, I was told I have hypertension at my company's health examination even though my blood pressure is usually within normal limits at home. What should I do, doctor? Do I have to start taking new medicine for hypertension?"

Actually, however, this type of hypertension is called "white coat syndrome," and is not serious in most case. Only when the patient is being examined in front of a doctor wearing a white coat does the patient's blood pressure rise. Such patients are often nervous and worried about having abnormal blood pressure, especially hypertension. In addition, because they strongly desire to get normal results in front of the physician, they tend to become more and more nervous.

On that day, I said the following three things to each patient individually

1: The fact that you feel nervous is quite natural. When you step in front of a doctor, you might feel uncomfortable, which will switch

on your sympathetic nervous system. As a result, your blood pressure will rise instinctively. This is a normal reaction. You don't need to feel nervous. In fact, I recommend that you just accept the phenomenon. Furthermore, try telling yourself (especially for a woman) "Oh, how pure-hearted and cute I am for getting nervous like this!"

2 : Breathe out deeply and slowly. Breathing out will switch on your parasympathetic nervous system and you will feel calm and relaxed.

3 : Massage your fingernails softly. This can also stimulate your parasympathetic nervous system.

Using these methods, you can be calm even in front of a doctor with a scary face.

However, if a patient still gets nervous during a blood pressure examination, I tell them just before the test: "Please TRY to raise your blood pressure as much as possible! You can do it!" Most patients laugh, "Oh, no, I can't, doctor. You must be joking again." As a result, their blood pressure decreases to a normal range.

As long as monitor your blood pressure regularly at home, and your results are normal, that's good enough. You should not worry about your blood pressure, even if it rises up temporarily during an examination.

However, we should be careful in such a case. There is always the chance that the patient's home measurements are wrong, and the doctor's result is actually correct (meaning that the patient truly has hypertension). We have to confirm which is actually the case and patients need to take regular measurements at the same time every day. Please check your blood pressure whenever you feel sick, have a headache, or feel anything abnormal. Record your results in your notebook. If you are worried whether your blood pressure monitor is working or not, please bring it to the clinic and show me how you usually use it at home. We can examine and compare your device with mine. Doing regular blood pressure examinations is a very good habit because it is non-invasive and not painful, yet very useful to detect a variety of diseases.

Additionally, please describe your first result in your notebook, when you examine your blood pressure at home. Some patients redo the examination again and again until they get an ideal figure, because they want to get a "perfect" to record. You don't have to do that. Please be honest and write down your first result each time, which will be more useful for evaluating your health.

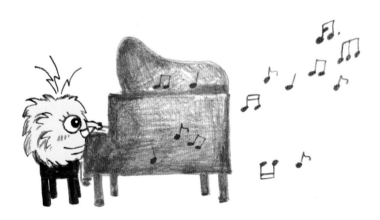

うつ病の治療に向けての説明

　うつ病患者さんに対して、私のクリニックでは、水力発電所のダムの水量
と発電機の様子に例えた4枚のボードを使って説明しています。
（香川大学　岡田宏基教授監修イラストより引用）

Let me illustrate the details of depression.

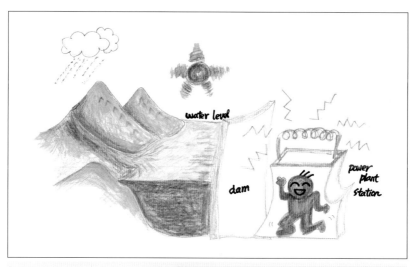

Picture 1

水位がちゃんと保たれたダムが元気で水力発電のできている発電機の様子

　Imagine there is a dam running a power plant station. If conditions
are normal, the dam is filled with enough water and the power
generator works smoothly (in this analogy, water symbolizes our
mental energy).

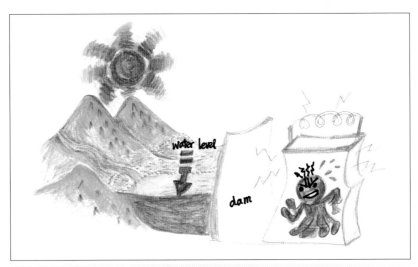

Picture 2

ダムの水位が下がっているのに、無理してさらにがむしゃらに働き続けている発電機の様子

If the generator continues to work without a replenishing water supply, the energy of the power station will gradually decrease because even without new water the generator is still continuing its work. Most depressive disorder patients repress in their true feelings of fatigue. This is very dangerous. People should listen to their bodies and minds carefully.

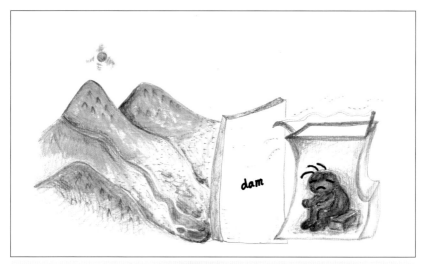

Picture 3

とうとうダムの水が枯れて、動けなくなって発電ができなくなった発電機の様子

Consequently, when the dam dries up, the generator can't work anymore. In these analogies, water represents our own energy, the lack of which leads to a depressive state.

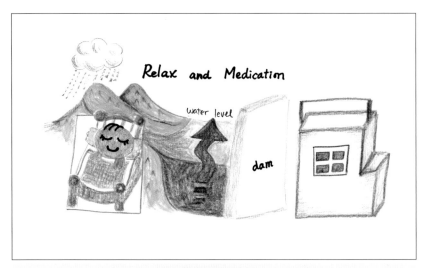

Picture 4

うつ病の治療には、休息と薬物療法が必要であるという図

In order to get better, you should try to find a place (and time) where you can reliably relax. Especially for most housewives, going to a hospital to take a rest is a good idea because they might be too distracted to relax at home. If you can feel at ease at home, you can take a rest there. If you decide to be an outpatient and stay at home with your family, please don't force yourself to do anything you don't want to do just because your family wants to make you join recreation activities and so on. Of course, if you want to participate, you should make the decision by yourself.

Antidepressant medication is very important, because the symptoms of depression are linked to functional issues involving neurotransmitters like serotonin. It will probably take three or four weeks for the effects of the anti-depressant to be felt. Only one dose will not be able to make you feel better immediately, but in three or four weeks you should start to feel better if the drugs are suitable for you. If not, we will try a different medication or dosage. Please try to relax, both mentally and physically, while we observe the effectiveness of the drugs.

If you have any questions, or something is not clear, please don't hesitate to ask me. I will be happy to explain further.

もし質問やわかりにくいところがあったら、どうぞ遠慮なさらずにお聞きになってくださいね。

付録
2

Questionnaire 質問用紙

Full Name :

Home Address :

Telephone number :

Date of birth :   /   /   (age   )

Nationality :

Gender :   male / female / other

How did you know about our clinic?

What is your chief health complaint? (What brings you here today?)

When did this problem begin?   /   /   (Year/ Month/ Day)

Have you ever had similar problem before?

Have you ever seen a psychiatrist or psychologist before?
                              (If yes, where?   )

Have you ever taken psychiatric medication?

Are you taking any medication now?

Have you ever had a serious health condition in the past?

　　他に何かありますか？ Anything else？ と尋ねましょう。まず
　　単数で聞いてから、他には？ と続けたほうが感じがいいようです。

資料：Himawari Mental Clinic Questionnaire『 大慌て！ 精神科医ひろこ先生の英語で診療・練習帳 』小林博子著（HOUSE出版）

Have you ever been injured in an accident?

Do you have any allergies?　　ここは複数形がいいようです。

Do you take any supplements?

Do you drink alcohol?　Yes / No
　　　　　　　　　　　Every day?　Just on occasion?
　　　　　　　　　　　How much?
　　　　　　　　　　　What kind of alcohol do you like best?

Do you smoke?　　　　Yes / No
　　　　　　　　　　　How many cigarettes do you smoke
　　　　　　　　　　　per day?

With whom do you live now?

Are you married?

Do you have children?　Yes / No
　　　　　　　　　　　How many?　How old are your children?

How tall are you?　(　　　　cm)

How much do you weigh?　(　　　kg)

Have you gained or lost weight recently?

What do you do for fun?

What country are you from?

How long have you lived in Japan?

What brought you to this country?（居住しているとき）

What brings you to this country?（旅行などのとき）

資料：Himawari Mental Clinic Questionnaire 『 大慌て！ 精神科医ひろこ先生の英語で診療・練習帳 』小林博子著（HOUSE出版）

Employment information

Place of work :

Employers（past and present）:
（Are you currently working at a job outside your home?）

Are you satisfied with your work?

Have you had any problems related to living in Japan?

Did you have any health or social problems in kindergarten?

Primary school?

Junior or high school?

College/ University?

Religion（voluntary question）

資料：Himawari Mental Clinic Questionnaire『 大慌て！ 精神科医ひろこ先生の英語で診療・練習帳 』小林博子著（HOUSE出版）

体について知っておきたい単語

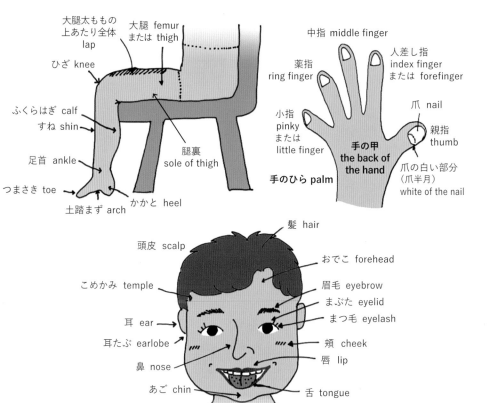

大腿太ももの上あたり全体 lap
大腿 femur または thigh
ひざ knee
ふくらはぎ calf
すね shin
足首 ankle
つまさき toe
土踏まず arch
腿裏 sole of thigh
かかと heel

中指 middle finger
薬指 ring finger
人差し指 index finger または forefinger
小指 pinky または little finger
爪 nail
親指 thumb
手の甲 the back of the hand
手のひら palm
爪の白い部分（爪半月）white of the nail

髪 hair
頭皮 scalp
こめかみ temple
耳 ear
耳たぶ earlobe
鼻 nose
あご chin
おでこ forehead
眉毛 eyebrow
まぶた eyelid
まつ毛 eyelash
頬 cheek
唇 lip
舌 tongue

	医学的には	一般的には
尿	urine	pee
糞便	feces / stool	poop
おなら	flatus	fart
しゃっくり	singultus	hiccup
げっぷする	belch	burp
あくび	oscitation	yawn

Bret先生からのお便り

Foreigners living in Japan face a variety of challenges. Of course, learning the language is first among these challenges, but there are many others: learning how to navigate train lines and subway systems, learning how to cook new foods, developing a new social network, finding a job, finding a place to live. The list goes on and on. Fortunately, most of these activities are enjoyable. I personally have never felt homesick. Japan is my home now.

However, the problem of getting good healthcare can be more daunting for foreigners—especially those new to the country. This might seem surprising. After all, Japan's doctors are knowledgeable and experienced. They have access to the world's best in medical equipment and pharmaceuticals. The national health insurance system ensures that anyone who needs treatment is eligible to receive it.

In spite of these positive aspects, many foreigners complain about such issues as the inability to make appointments, which leads to excessively long waiting times. Most are also shocked at the very short amount of time they are given to actually consult with the doctor. Dosage recommendations can be a source of concern when they are different from what would be expected in the patient's home country. And the prospect of having to ride an ambulance can be downright terrifying!

Many foreigners have resorted to various "workarounds" such as trying to have medications sent to them from relatives abroad (the legality of which is often questionable). Some will only go the hospital if absolutely necessary. One word of advice that circulates in the expatriate community is to never call an ambulance because you never know how long the ride will take or what hospital you will be taken to. Instead, one should call a taxi and go to your preferred hospital. The reasoning is that if you do somehow manage to stumble up to the reception desk, at least the hospital won't be able to refuse you care!

Obviously, such workarounds are not ideal. Most of them could be overcome, or at least improved, through better doctor/patient communication. Certainly, the main responsibility for language acquisition lies with the newcomer to Japan. That said, learning Japanese is a time-consuming process and very difficult for some. It is for this reason that I was pleased to assist Dr. Hiroko in producing the present volume. Her dedication to her patients and to the practice of medicine itself is evident on every page. I sincerely hope Dr. Hiroko's enthusiasm and efforts will be inspirational to others working in the medical field. **Bret Fisk**

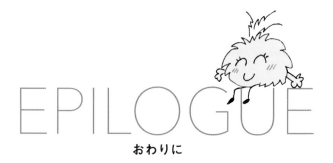

EPILOGUE

おわりに

　いかがでしたか？

　もしも日本語を母国語としない患者さんが、英語で日本の医療機関にかかるとしたら、それは大変勇気のいることだと思います。ましてや、精神科へなんて、すごく大変なことだろうと思います。そういった患者さんたちが日本で少しでも心地よく幸せに過ごしていけるように、何とかお手伝いしていきたいと思っています。英語を母国語とする方々でも、国により、地方により、発音や伝え方が違ったりするでしょうし、また、ほかの国のご出身で国際語として英語を習得された方でも、標準となる言い回しと違う表現をされる患者さんも多いかと思います。

　やはり、そんなときには、「習うより慣れろ」なのかもしれませんね。いろいろ話してみて、やってみて、時には誤解のないように筆談したりして、丁寧に信頼関係を築きながら、対応していくのがいいのだろうと思います。

　私はこの本をお守りとして脇に携えながら、怖がらずに頑張っていきたいと思います。そして、いつか、この本がどなたかほかの方の役に立てればうれしいです。読んでいただきありがとうございました。また、丁寧に添削してくださったブレット先生に、多大なる感謝を申し上げます。

ひまわりメンタルクリニック院長　小林博子

Thank you for reading this book through to the very end.
Did you enjoy it? I hope your answer is "YES!"

Anybody can easily understand how it must be very difficult and require courage for foreigners, who don't speak Japanese yet, to decide to go to a Japanese hospital, when they feel sick especially regarding mental health. We should all try to help them be as comfortable and happy as possible in Japanese clinics and hospitals.

This book is written in English, but there are a lot of differences of pronunciation or dialect even within the English-speaking countries such as Australia, New Zealand, Canada, the UK and the US. Still more patients from other countries who have learned English as a second language will have their own challenges when trying to express their feelings in English. Although it must be difficult for me to see foreign patients, I know the day will come when I will have to treat them. I can only hope that with experience I can give them the best care possible. Preparation is everything, and only practice gives us exceptional advice and makes our skills improve. I'm sure I will have to talk a lot with these patients, and sometimes we may even need to communicate in writing or drawing in order to build a relationship of trust with each other.

I will always keep this book beside me to be my lifesaver, when I see patients in English. It is my hope that this book will be of benefit for other doctors like me. I really wish the best for all patients and doctors in Japan.

I'm very grateful to Bret Fisk for giving me much helpful and encouraging advice with this book. I couldn't have done it without him.

Dr. Hiroko Kobayashi, M.D. Himawari Mental Clinic

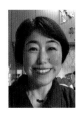

著者　小林博子（こばやし・ひろこ）
HIROKO KOBAYASHI , M. D .

ひまわりメンタルクリニック院長。横浜市立大学医学部卒業、
同大学大学院医学研究科博士課程修了。医学博士。精神保健
指定医、老年精神医学専門医、認知症サポート医。「小田原・
箱根・湯河原・真鶴一市三町若年性認知症を考える会」代表

ひまわりメンタルクリニック
http://www.asahi-net.or.jp/~an7h-kbys/

デザイン　峯岸孝之（COMIX BRAND）
編集　　　早川景子

大慌て! 精神科医ひろこ先生の英語で診療・練習帳
A Psychiatrist's English Training Manual

2021年12月24日　初版　第1刷発行
著　者　小林博子
発行者　内門大丈
発行所　HOUSE出版株式会社
〒254-0046 神奈川県平塚市立野町28-27
電話 0463-71-6141
印刷・製本所　藤原印刷株式会社